Clinical Aspects of Inhaled Particles

Clinical Aspects of Inhaled Particles

Edited by **D. C. F. Muir,** *PhD MRCP*

Head of Physiology Branch, Institute of Occupational Medicine, Edinburgh
Hon. Consultant Physician, City Hospital, Edinburgh

William Heinemann Medical Books Limited
London

First Published 1972

ISBN: 0 433 28200 2

Text set in 10/11 pt. Monotype Times New Roman, printed by letterpress, and bound in Great Britain at The Pitman Press, Bath

CONTRIBUTORS

P. Lesley Bidstrup, MD FRCP FRACCP, Clinical Assistant, Chest Department, St. Thomas's Hospital, London; Formerly Assistant, Department for Research in Industrial Medicine, Medical Research Council.

P. C. Elmes, MD FRCP, Whitla Professor of Therapeutics and Pharmacology, The Queen's University of Belfast.

P. J. Lawther, MB DSc FRCP, Director of the MRC Air Pollution Unit, Professor of Environmental Medicine at St. Bartholomew's Hospital Medical College and Physician-in-Charge of the Department of Preventive and Environmental Medicine at St. Bartholomew's Hospital, London.

C. B. McKerrow, MD FRCP, Member of the Scientific Staff, Medical Research Council Pneumoconiosis Unit, Penarth.

D. C. F. Muir, PhD MRCP, Head of Physiology Branch, Institute of Occupational Medicine, Edinburgh; Hon. Consultant Physician, City Hospital, Edinburgh.

R. S. F. Schilling, MD DSc FRCP DPh DIH, Director of the TUC Centenary Institute of Occupational Health, London; Professor of Occupational Health, London School of Hygiene and Tropical Medicine.

R. E. O. Williams, MD FRCP FRCPath, Professor of Bacteriology, St. Mary's Hospital Medical School, London.

Foreword

Most patients suffering from disease of the respiratory tract contracted their illness as a result of inhaling airborne particles of one type or another. Diseases caused in this way include chronic bronchitis and carcinoma of the bronchus due to tobacco smoke or urban air pollution and allergic reactions such as hay fever, asthma or alveolitis. Tuberculosis and other infections may gain access to the body through the respiratory tract and there are many industrial dusts which can cause pulmonary disease. Many of these same patients are subsequently treated by means of therapeutic aerosols.

The interaction of inhaled particles and the lungs is thus a major factor in the pathogenesis of respiratory disease and in its treatment. In collecting these reviews by different authors every effort has been made to assemble information concerning the physical properties of the airborne material and to relate its behaviour in the lung to the resulting disease. Attention is directed to those aspects of interest to the practising clinician, and radioactive aerosols are therefore omitted since they are highly specialized and, it is hoped, will not be encountered in clinical practice. The systemic effects of airborne toxins are not considered for the same reasons.

No attempt has been made to make this a comprehensive reference work on current aerosol research since this changes too rapidly. However, the general pattern changes more slowly and the book is intended to present a broad view of the effects of inhaled particles on the lung.

March 1972 D. C. F. MUIR

Contents

Page

Chapter 1

Deposition and Clearance of Inhaled Particles

D. C. F. MUIR

The average human subject inhales approximately 10,000 litres of air each day. This air contains a great deal of suspended particulate matter, some of which is deposited in the lung and the remainder exhaled. The effect of this dust on the health of the individual depends on the nature of the particles and on the site of their deposition in the respiratory tract. In order to understand the nature of this process it is necessary to understand the physical laws governing the motion of airborne particles, the anatomy of the lung and the pattern of airflow during breathing. Current ideas on the behaviour of particles in the lungs are probably fairly accurate although it is not yet possible to obtain direct experimental proof of all the details.

Definition of an Aerosol

Various names are used to describe airborne particles. Dusts, mists, smokes, fumes and fog are familiar terms and have certain technical meanings. The word aerosol is a general name referring to any atmosphere containing particles which remain airborne for a reasonable length of term and is used to describe all particles than can be inhaled whether they are therapeutic, industrial, or of natural origin such as bacteria, fungi and pollens.

Deposition of Aerosol Particles in the Lung

As inhaled particles enter the respiratory tract with each inspiration they closely follow the moving airstreams. In addition, they possess a limited mobility independent of the airflow which may cause a certain proportion to come into contact with the wall of the airway. A particle which has once touched any portion of the surface of the lung in this way cannot be resuspended by the airflows which are normally encountered and is thus filtered or deposited from the air. Each particle behaves as an independent unit and, within limits, the actual number concentration is unimportant.

The motion of particles which results in deposition is related to their size, density and shape. It does not depend on their composition or on whether they are in a solid or liquid state. Although therapeutic aerosols and some fungal spores consist of round particles, many industrial dusts have irregular shapes and may be clumped together in loose aggregates. The behaviour of such complex particles is best understood by first describing the factors causing spherical particles to move towards the surface of the airway and to result in their deposition. Three independent mechanisms may be distinguished—

(1) **Sedimentation.** All particles suspended in a gas slowly sediment under the influence of gravity. The effects of the viscosity of the surrounding gas is such that each particle falls at a constant speed. This speed (the terminal velocity) is proportional to the density of the particle and to the square of its diameter. Large particles fall considerably faster than small ones and a particle of silica or iron falls faster than a pollen grain of the same size. The simple relation of terminal velocity to particle density and diameter is constant for most aerosols of clinical interest but special corrections must be made for particles with diameters greater than about 20 μ and for those with diameters smaller than 1 μ.

(2) **Diffusion.** Airborne particles are continuously subjected to bombardment by the surrounding gas molecules. This induces a random movement of the particles called Brownian motion which results in their transfer or diffusion from one region of a gas volume to another. The diffusivity of a particle is inversely proportional to its diameter but is independent of its density. Very small particles diffuse rapidly although the rate of their diffusion is orders of magnitude below that of gases. Both diffusivity and sedimentation have very low values for particles with diameters of about 0·5 μ; as a result they follow any movement of the surrounding air very closely indeed.

(3) **Inertia.** If the direction of airflow changes then the inertia of any suspended particles causes them to continue in the original direction for a certain distance, depending on the velocity and angle of change in direction of the airstream, and, as does its terminal velocity, on the density of the particle and square of its diameter.

Gravitational settlement or sedimentation causes particle deposition only on the lower surfaces of the airways or alveoli but diffusion is a random process causing very small particles to be deposited on all surfaces. Inertial movement causes deposition or impaction on the opposing wall of the airway. For a given velocity of airflow it causes a greater fraction of particles to be impacted in smaller airways where the particles are, on average, closer to the wall. The eddy motion of turbulent airflow in the trachea also causes some deposition of large particles in this region.

The branching pattern of the bronchial tree has two outstanding features which influence the nature of airflow in the lung and the deposition of inhaled particles. In the first place the diameter of the airways becomes progressively smaller with each successive division. The major bronchi have diameters of about 1 cm while the respiratory bronchioles and alveolar ducts have diameters of only about 1 mm. The chances of a particle being deposited in a given time due to diffusion or sedimentation are much higher in a small airway than in the major bronchi since it has a greater chance of reaching the boundary wall if it has less distance to travel and the probability of it being deposited by these two mechanisms therefore increases as it is drawn further into the lung.

The second feature is a result of the increase in the total number of airways with each division. Although the calibre of the airways in the depths of the lungs is so small their number is enormous and the total cross sectional area correspondingly large. A given volume of air thus moves more and more slowly as it passes further into the lung. While the high speed of airflow causes significant impaction of particles in the nose and larger bronchi the reduction in impaction efficiency due to the low air velocity in small airways is balanced to some extent by their small calibre and the fraction of particles entering the tenth generation of airways which is removed by impaction is similar to that removed in the third generation.

The concept of the filtration efficiency of the airways of the lung has been familiar for many years and was first noted by Lister (1868). He observed that penetrating wounds of the chest frequently gave rise to an infected pneumothorax but that this complication was unusual when the air entered the pleural cavity from the lung, as in a spontaneous pneumothorax. He surmised that the difference was due to the removal of bacteria from the air as it passed down the airways. Tyndall (1870) demonstrated that light was not scattered from air exhaled from the deep parts of the lung and concluded that floating matter was not present in the air of these regions but had been filtered out. Owens (1923) repeated these experiments and showed that deep lung air did contain dust particles following a maximal inhalation but was free of dust following a period of quiet breathing. He suggested that "during quiet breathing, the air drawn in does not reach the alveoli, and the interchange which takes place between the inspired air and that already in the lungs is mainly by diffusion, with some light mechanical mixing at the points of contact". He thought that particles were unlikely to be carried beyond the cilia under resting conditions and that this was an important factor in maintaining the health of the subject. His ideas have turned out to be close to the truth.

Findeisen (1935) first examined the relationship between the mobility of the particles, the calibre of the airways and the speed of airflow in each region. He was able to calculate the total deposition of particles in the lung and the actual site of their deposition. Although there were some errors in his calculations his general conclusions were valid. He showed that large particles are completely filtered out of the inhaled air by means of gravitational sedimentation or by impaction and that all the very small particles are also deposited as a result of their high diffusion coefficient. A proportion of the particles in the middle range are deposited but a considerable fraction escape deposition and are exhaled. Particles of about 0·5 μ diameter have the least probability of being deposited. He estimated the fraction of inhaled particles deposited in each region of the lung by considering the effectiveness of the deposition mechanism in each airway. He showed that the high mobility of very large and of very small particles results in their deposition high in the respiratory tract and that they have very little chance of penetrating to the alveolar regions. Although the total deposition of the more stable aerosols in the middle range is small they have a greater net deposition within the alveoli.

An analysis of this type presents considerable difficulties. The essential feature is to consider the lung to be composed of a series of filters constituted by the different airways. A given volume of inhaled air is then supposed to consist of separate small fractions, each of which passes a certain distance into the lung depending on its position within the whole volume of inhaled air. The time that a particle spends in each region of the lung is then calculated from a knowledge of the rate of breathing, the total cross sectional area of the airways at any given point and the length of each airway. Appropriate calculations are made for each bifurcation to estimate the effects of impaction. Landahl (1950) improved upon Findeisen's method and his results formed the basis of a more detailed analysis by Beeckmans (1965).

Several mathematical approximations are made in these calculations and a number of assumptions made about the physiology of the lung. Accurate descriptions of the morphology of the lung have only recently become available and the detailed behaviour of the moving airstreams is still not understood. Some reservation must, therefore, be made about our ability to predict the site of particle deposition in the lung. There is difficulty in determining the exact distribution of inhaled air. As was first pointed out by Owens (1923) the volume of each inspiration is important since particles can only penetrate into the lung if they are transported there by the mass movement of air. A greater fraction of each inhalation reaches the alveolar region of the lung if the tidal volume is increased but the relationship is by no means straightforward. Although the airflow in the trachea is turbulent it has been suggested that the tidal air in the small airways advances with a cone shaped front as a result of the velocity gradients present in laminar flow and that this causes particles to penetrate into the alveolar ducts a good deal further than comparison between the volume of inhaled air and that of the airways would suggest. Present evidence on the nature of airflow in the lung indicates that this simplification is unlikely to be realized in practice. The disturbance of flow produced by the repetitive branching pattern of the airway mitigates against the establishment of the velocity gradients necessary for the development of a cone shaped interface between the tidal air and the lung air.

The duration of each breath is important because it determines the fraction of particles deposited by sedimentation or diffusion during that breath. For a given minute ventilation rapid shallow breathing reduces the overall particle deposition and, in particular, reduces the fraction of aerosol penetrating to the alveoli. On the other hand, slow deep breathing increases the deposition of aerosol in the depths of the lung and this pattern of breathing is often used in the administration of therapeutic substances. Deposition due to impaction is unaffected by the depth or frequency of breathing at a fixed minute ventilation since it is a function only of the mean rate of airflow.

The minute ventilation, rate of breathing and tidal volume all increase on exercise. Although this reduces the time for sedimentation and diffusion to result in particle deposition during each breath the higher mean rate of airflow causes more efficient impaction of particles and the larger tidal volume draws the aerosol further into the smaller airways of the lung. The fractional deposition of inhaled aerosols therefore probably remains fairly constant in the resting or exercising subject and this has been confirmed experimentally by Muir and Davies (1967) in the case of 0·5 μ diameter particles. The total dose of material absorbed by the resting or exercising subject is therefore directly proportional to the minute ventilation.

Total deposition of aerosol in the lung can be measured by experiment and a number of studies have been published (Drinker *et al.*, 1928; Brown, 1931; Van Wijk and Patterson, 1940; Landahl and Herrmann, 1948; Brown *et al.*, 1950; Landahl *et al.*, 1952; Altshuler *et al.*, 1957; Dautrebande *et al.*, 1957; Muir and Davies, 1967; Dennis, 1961). The wide range of the experimental results is an outstanding feature of these reports. Brown *et al.* (1950) for example found that about 35% of particles with diameters of 0·5 μ were deposited in the lung during breathing while Muir and Davies (1967) reported values of only 15%. The various results were obtained by widely different techniques but all based on the general principle of measuring the total amount of aerosol inhaled, the amount exhaled and of calculating the amount deposited by simple subtraction. Much confusion has arisen because of failure to distinguish between the effects of changes in the rate of breathing from those associated with changes in the depth of breathing. An experimental subject who is instructed to breathe slowly at rest usually breathes more deeply so that his minute volume remains relatively constant. Under these conditions it is not possible to be certain whether any changes in particle deposition are the result of changes in the rate or in the depth of breathing. The experiments of

Muir and Davies (1967) separated these factors but they studied a single particle size only.

Experiments of this type do not give direct information about the regional deposition of particles in the lung. Brown *et al.* (1950) tackled the problem by measuring the concentration of particles in different fractions of exhaled air. They measured the carbon dioxide concentration of the air at the same time and used this as an indication of the origin of the exhaled particles. Aerosol contained in air with a high carbon dioxide content was assumed to have come from the alveolar region of the lung. From this information they calculated the fraction of inhaled particles that had been deposited in the alveoli. The difficulty of this approach is that we do not really know the origin of the particles in any given fraction of exhaled air. A single particle in the air may have travelled from the depths of the lung in a rapidly moving axial airstream or may equally have been carried by a slowly moving stream from the periphery of a large airway. Gas concentrations can give only a very approximate indication of the origin of airborne particles because of the rapid diffusion of molecules which results in a more efficient washout of the dead space gas than is possible with aerosols. The assymetrical nature of the bronchial tree presents further problems since Horsfield and Cumming (1968) have shown that a given fraction of exhalate contains contributions of alveolar air from regions with short path lengths together with air from the upper airways of regions with longer pathways.

Altshuler (1959) and Altshuler *et al.* (1967) developed the most complete theory relating the concentration of aerosol in exhaled air to the regional deposition of particles. The possible factors outlined above were considered in detail and allowances made so that suitable adjustments can be made to the model as further data regarding airflow in the lung is established.

Indirect evidence on the site of particle deposition in the lung can be obtained by post mortem examination of lung dust and by radioactive techniques in man or by experiments in animals. These are discussed in the section on retention of dust in the lung.

Aerosol Deposition in the Nose

Early accounts underestimated the importance of particle deposition in the nose. Although it is difficult to allow for the irregular shape of the nasal cavities, Landahl (1950) showed by calculation and subsequent experiment that the nose is a major site of particle deposition. Few particles greater than 20 μ in diameter and only about 50% of particles of 5 μ in diameter are able to penetrate the nose during breathing at rest. Proctor *et al.* (1969) have shown that many particles even as small as 1 μ in diameter are deposited in the nose during normal breathing and that much of this is on the unciliated anterior portion of the nose.

Proctor and Swift (1971) have pointed out that the nose is probably of about the same efficiency as a filter as are the ciliated airways themselves. A particle which does manage to penetrate the nose is thus likely to be carried right through to the alveoli. It is of interest to note that, by tradition, many coal miners in Britain chew tobacco with the deliberate intention of forcing themselves to breathe through the nose. Their supposition that this may protect their lungs is probably well founded.

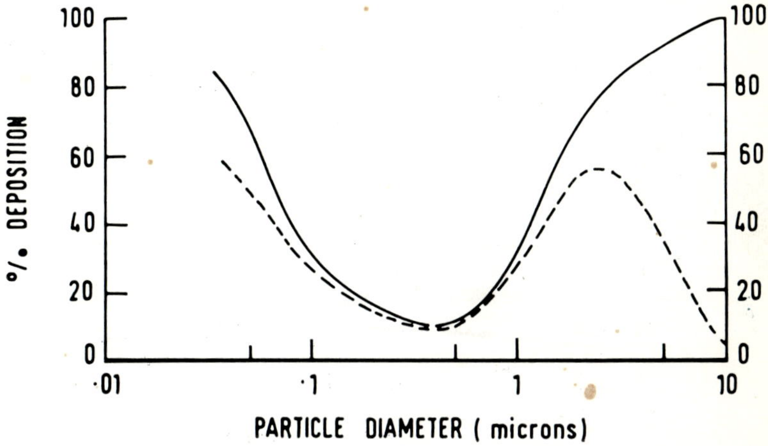

FIG. 1. Per cent deposition of inhaled aerosols as a function of particle size. Mouth breathing at rest. Total deposition (——) alveolar deposition (----).

The method of breathing must be considered in assessing the direct relevance of laboratory experiments to industrial practice. Many experiments are carried out with mouth breathing although most working subjects only do so on fairly heavy exercise or when speaking.

Total and Alveolar Deposition of Particles: Respirable Dust

From the practical point of view it is important to know both the total deposition of inhaled particles of various sizes and, in particular, the proportion which is deposited beyond the terminal bronchiole—the so-called alveolar or respirable dust. This dust is of special importance because it is associated with the development of pneumoconiosis. An illustration of the total and alveolar deposition of inhaled particles is shown in Fig. 1. Fractional deposition in the nose, ciliated airways and alveoli is shown in Fig. 2 which is based on all the evidence available up to 1966 and which was reviewed by a task group of the International Commission on Radiological Protection. There is disagreement as to the size of particle at which alveolar deposition is maximum. Wide acceptance has been given to the results of Brown *et al.* (1950) who suggested that it was about 1 μ, and this size is favoured by Davies (1964). Other authors have calculated that it lies between 2 μ and 4 μ. (Findeisen, 1935; Landahl, 1950; Beeckmans, 1965; Altshuler *et al.*, 1967).

Particle Shape: Aggregation: Aerodynamic Size

The deposition of dust in the lung depends on the sedimentation, impaction and diffusion of the individual particles which, if they are

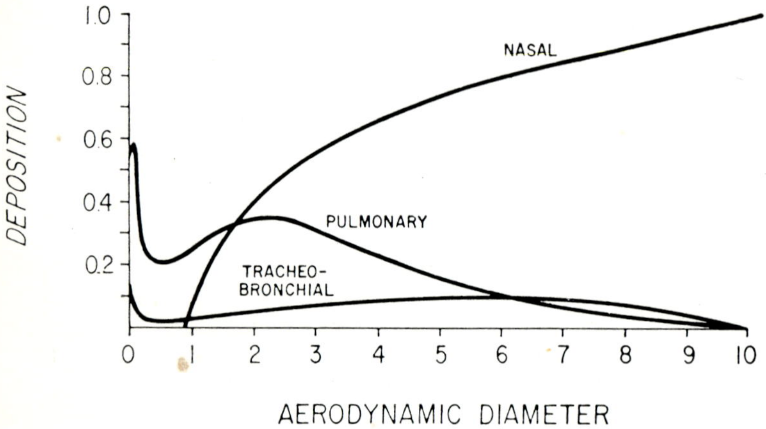

FIG. 2. Regional deposition of inhaled aerosols as a function of particle size (μ). Nose breathing at 15 respirations per minute and 750 cm³ tidal volume. The pulmonary compartment refers to deposition beyond the terminal bronchiole.
(Reproduced from *Health Physics*, **12**, 179 (1966) by permission of the Health Physics Society.)

spherical, are functions of their diameters. However most dust in industry is of irregular shape and may be aggregated into loose clumps. The behaviour of such dusts depends entirely on the mobility or settling velocity of the particles or aggregates and not on their apparent microscopic size. A clump of coal dust may thus appear to be some 15 μ in diameter but, if its structure is fairly loose, it may only sediment with the same speed as a 7 μ diameter sphere. When inhaled into the lung it will therefore be deposited in the same manner as if it were a 7 μ diameter sphere. The behaviour of the particle is most easily described by stating the size of sphere of unit density which has the same terminal velocity and which will thus have an identical intrapulmonary deposition pattern. The aerodynamic size, or diameter of the equivalent unit density sphere (EUDS) of the above mentioned 15 μ diameter coal dust particle is thus 7 μ.

Clearance of Dust From the Lung: Dust Retention

Soluble substances are rapidly absorbed from all regions of the respiratory tract. Insoluble particles which land on the ciliated epithelium are transported to the pharynx and are then swallowed or expectorated. The rate of clearance by the cilia is independent of the size of the particles on its surface and of their concentration, unless they have some specific toxic action. However, large particles are deposited high in the respiratory tract while those of smaller size are able to penetrate nearer to the terminal bronchiole. The latter are, therefore, cleared more slowly because they must traverse a greater distance along the mucosa and, in this sense only, does the rate of ciliary clearance depend on the size of the particle.

The rate of ciliary clearance has been extensively studied in man by means of radioactive aerosols and by using external scintillation counters. The clearance of the healthy mucosa is essentially complete in less than 24 hours. Most of the dust trapped on the mucosa of a man working in a dusty trade is cleared before the next day's shift and it does not accumulate during regular daily work.

Dust depositing in the alveolus is cleared very much more slowly. Within a few hours of deposition it is engulfed by the alveolar macrophages. Non toxic dusts are subsequently carried by the macrophages towards the ciliated epithelium where they are excreted by the mucous escalator. The macrophage response appears to be a mechanism for the protection of the alveolar epithelium which probably cannot be penetrated by particles if they are within phagocytes. The rate of the clearance mechanism has been studied by brief exposure of animals or human volunteers to low concentrations of dust labelled with radioactive tracers. Alveolar clearance under these experimental conditions is approximately exponential with respect to time and has a half life of about 60–120 days. There is uncertainty about the amount of dust which is cleared from the lung during daily exposure in industry. If the fractional deposition values shown in Figs. 1 and 2 are correct, then a coalminer working under poor conditions may receive a total alveolar dust load of something like 1,000 g during a life time of work. Despite this high figure it is unusual to find more than about 40 g of dust in the lungs of miners at post mortem examination. These figures suggest that the alveolar clearance mechanism is highly efficient. An alternative explanation is to suppose that the alveolar clearance is less efficient but that the initial rate of particle deposition within the alveolus is much lower than has previously been thought (Davies, 1967). There is certainly much experimental work to support the suggestion that alveolar clearance of dust following chronic exposure is a relatively slow process (Stöber, Einbrodt and Klosterkötter, 1967; Klosterkötter and Bünemann, 1961; Le Bouffant, 1961). Experimental work with animals has shown that the rate of alveolar clearance is proportional to the total amount of dust in the lungs, provided that the initial burden is not too great. The rate is probably related to the availability of macrophages whose number increases in response to an alveolar dust load (Brain, 1971) and the removal of the foreign matter is thus facilitated. There is some evidence that this is also true in the case of human exposure. Dust does not appear to accumulate in the lungs of miners at a steady rate and the amount of dust in the lungs at any given time is not simply a function of the total number of days or years of exposure. It was shown to rise fairly rapidly during the first ten years or so and then to level off or rise much more slowly by Stöber *et al.* (1967) whose findings were based on post mortem examination of the lungs of miners and on their occupational exposure during life. However, very little accurate information of long term individual exposure is usually available and more studies of this type are required.

The amount of dust in the lung at any instant, the dust retention, represents a balance between the rate of its accumulation from the tidal air and the rate of its subsequent removal. Some penetrates through the alveolar wall, and is retained permanently in the lymphatics and hilar lymph glands. When it is in the tissues it is usually contained within macrophages although this does not imply that it penetrates the alveolar wall in the free state (Schiller, 1961). Cytotoxic dusts such as quartz have a particularly marked tendency to penetrate the alveolar wall and to accumulate in the lung. The particles in lung dust are not static and Heppleston (1961) was able to demonstrate a progressive intermingling of particles in the lungs of rats exposed to two different non-fibrogenic dusts on different occasions separated by an interval of up to six months. This intermingling took place throughout the pulmonary dust foci and also within individual macrophages. The process is best explained by the repeated death of grossly laden cells with liberation of their dust and its subsequent ingestion by fresh generations of macrophages. In coal workers, the dust is found round the respiratory bronchioles in depots containing particles which had been deposited, in the first instance, throughout the alveoli and which were then transported by macrophages while still within the air space and packed into the alveoli opening off the respiratory bronchioles. These are eventually sealed off by epithelium and are no longer in communication with the air space (Heppleston, 1961).

The size distribution of lung dust was examined by McRae (1913) who noted that most of the particles in the lungs of rock miners were below 1 μ in diameter. The dust was very much finer than that in the inhaled air and it was correctly concluded that only fairly small particles could cause pneumoconiosis. By comparing the size distribution of the lung dust and of the airborne dust, Davies (1964) has estimated the fractional deposition of inhaled particles. Unfortunately it is not possible to be certain of the aerodynamic size of the aggregates in which many of the fine particles entered the respiratory tract. There is also evidence (Holma, 1967) that large particles are removed preferentially by the macrophage system and that the composition of the particles also determines the rate at which alveolar dust is taken up by macrophages. He found, for example, that carbon particles were ingested by macrophages much more avidly than polystyrene spheres of the same diameter. It is therefore highly likely that the size distribution and composition of alveolar dust changes with time and cannot be a reliable guide to the characteristics of the dust originally deposited in the lung.

The widely differing rates of alveolar and ciliary clearance have been used by Lippman and Albert (1969) to estimate the deposition of particles in each region. By assuming that clearance from the lungs of volunteer subjects within twenty-four hours of exposure to radioactive aerosols represented material initially deposited on the cilia, it was possible to calculate the fraction of the inhaled cloud which had penetrated to the alveoli. This work is still in progress and should give important information.

Non-uniform Aerosols: Mass Median Diameter

Most industrial dusts contain particles of a wide range of sizes and the fraction in each range must be measured before the intrapulmonary deposition of the whole cloud can be predicted in detail. Since the larger particles in such a cloud often contain the bulk of the airborne material the mean particle size or diameter of a mixed aerosol may give little indication of its effective distribution in the lung. This is particularly important in the case of therapeutic aerosols where a given spray may be stated to have a small mean droplet size. While this may be strictly true the therapeutic effect may, in fact, be determined by the presence of a relatively few large drops. Mixed clouds of this type should be characterized by determining the mass median diameter (MMD) which is that size where half the weight of the cloud is contained in particles larger than the stated size and half in smaller particles. Most natural aerosols have a skew or log normal distribution with an excess of small particles but the spread of sizes, or geometric standard deviation is usually within a fairly narrow range. As a result the deposition of non uniform dusts in each compartment of the lung can usually be expressed in terms of the MMD of the cloud and this is illustrated in Fig. 3. Size selective sampling instruments are now available which permit the MMD of an aerosol to be determined fairly easily. For specific industrial requirements selective sampling instruments have been designed which allow the respirable dust to be collected separately and these are now widely used for measuring the dust in British Coal Mines. They are provided with a pre-filter which removes the larger particles but which allows a fraction of the finer dust to penetrate and to be collected on a glass fibre filter for subsequent weighing and compositional analysis.

The sample includes all the airborne particles with an aerodynamic diameter of 1 μ, 50% of those of 5 μ diameter but none larger than 7 μ. That dust measurements based on this size distribution represent a

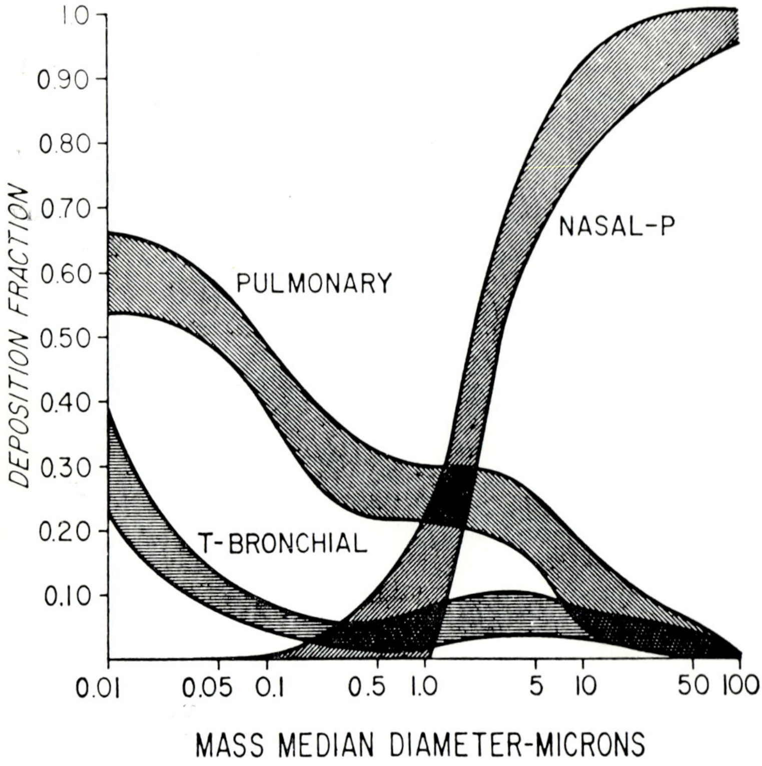

FIG. 3. Regional deposition of inhaled aerosols as a function of the mass median aerodynamic diameter of the cloud. Nose breathing with tidal volume of 1450 ml. The shaded areas include the ranges of cloud uniformity likely to be encountered in practice.
(Reproduced from the *Health Physics*. **12,** 181 (1966) by permission of the Health Physics Society.)

true measure of the risks to coalminers of developing simple pneumoconiosis has now been confirmed by the findings of Jacobsen *et al.* (1971).

Regional Distribution of Inhaled Particles

The ventilation of the lower zones of the lung of the upright resting subject is greater than that of the upper zones (West, 1965). While the initial distribution of inhaled aerosols almost certainly follows this general pattern it is a common feature of any post mortem examination that it is the apices of the upper lobes which are so heavily pigmented in city dwellers. The nature of this pigment has not been identified with certainty but it is clearly the result of inhaling polluted air. The fibrosis associated with coalworkers pneumoconiosis, silicosis and allergic alveolitis also tends to affect the upper lobes in particular. These conditions reflect the balance between the regional deposition of particles and the rate of their subsequent removal. While no information is available regarding the rate of alveolar clearance from different regions of the lung there is some evidence that the amount of dust in the upper lobes of coalminers is greater than in the lower lobes (Einbrodt, 1967) although asbestos particles are uniformly distributed throughout the lung (Bell and Elmes, 1968). If coal dust does accumulate in the upper lobes despite a greater initial deposition in the lower lobes then presumably clearance must be considerably slower from the former.

The distribution of particle deposition within the acinus itself is unknown. The proximal alveoli within the acinus are probably exposed to a higher concentration of aerosol than the distal units because each inhalation transports the particles to this point. Particles can only reach the terminal alveoli by the mechanical mixing of air in the lung described by Altshuler *et al.* (1959). Heppleston (1963) noted that the distribution of an experimental dust in rat lungs was very irregular and that some alveoli contained many particles, while adjacent and apparently identical alveoli, were completely clear.

Individual Variation: Effect of Smoking and of Lung Disease

Lehmann (1935) was the first to consider individual variations in the filtration efficiency of the airways as a causative factor in pneumoconiosis, although he was unable to find such evidence from experimental work on the nasal filtration of particles. Altshuler *et al.* (1957) showed clear differences between the pattern of deposition of inhaled particles in three normal subjects during mouth breathing. The rate of deposition appeared to be related to the amount of mechanical mixing of air in the lung and was evident when aerosols of various sizes were used. Love *et al.* (1971) carried out a detailed investigation of this problem. The fractional deposition of 1 μ diameter particles in the lungs was measured in 18 coal workers with Category II simple pneumoconiosis and in 40 control miners whose chest X-rays were normal. The two groups were carefully matched for age and occupational history. The deposition characteristics of the two groups were compared after standardizing for the tidal volume and frequency of breathing. No significant differences were found. It was concluded that individual variations in the deposition pattern were unlikely to be an important factor in causing the development of simple pneumoconiosis in coal-workers and that the disease, at this stage, was not associated with an increased dust deposition pattern. This latter finding is important because Jacobsen *et al.* (1971) have shown that the X-ray changes of simple pneumoconiosis appear to progress at a faster rate once the initial stages have developed.

Le Bouffant (1961) noted wide variations in the rates of alveolar clearance in rats although Wright (1961) pointed out that these are not observed during long term exposure experiments. There is no information on the range of alveolar clearance rate in man, although delayed clearance might well be an important factor in determining individual susceptibility to pneumoconiosis. Wide variations in the rate of bronchial clearance have been found in human experiments (Lipmann and Albert, 1969), and Lipmann, Albert and Peterson (1971) found that airway obstruction due to asthma or bronchitis increased the fraction of particles trapped in the larger airways. Sanchis *et al.* (1971) also found that less aerosol was able to penetrate to the alveoli in smokers compared with non-smokers, although they considered that this was due to small airway damage and could not be to the long term benefit of a miner. They found that the rate of ciliary clearance was impaired in smokers although no difference was found by Thomson and Short (1969).

This recent work on the interaction of dust and disease in the lung strongly suggests that the diseased lung cannot handle inhaled dust in the normal manner and appears to confirm J. T. Arlidge's advice in 1892 that "persons pre-disposed to respiratory diseases and phthisis ought not to engage in dusty occupations".

Change in Particle Size During Breathing

Hygroscopic substances such as sodium chloride, glycerine and some fractions of tobacco smoke rapidly absorb moisture as they enter the respiratory tract. On the other hand volatile substances may evaporate and, in each case, the associated change in the size and aerodynamic properties of the particles may radically alter their intrapulmonary deposition pattern. Therapeutic aerosols, droplet nuclei (see Chapter 3) and some types of fungal spore are affected in the same way. The stability of water droplets in the lung is discussed in Chapter 9.

Electrostatic Charge

The behaviour of inhaled aerosols is altered by the presence of an electrostatic charge on the particles. If each carries the same charge they repel each other towards the wall of the airway and this has the effect of increasing the overall deposition of particles in the lung but may reduce the number reaching the small airways. The airways themselves, being inside an electrically conducting body, are uncharged other than by induction from charged particles within the airway and an electric charge on the body cannot in itself influence the behaviour of particles once they have been inhaled. However, the body surface may be raised to a high potential when a subject inhales a cloud of charged particles and the charge is concentrated over pointed parts of the body such as the nose. This localized potential may repel further dust particles if they have the same polarity and prevent them entering the nose during breathing. The change in the deposition pattern produced by an electrostatic charge on the particles in a therapeutic aerosol is of no benefit to the patient and there is no evidence that the electric itself has any effect on the body. Many claims have been made for the clinical effectiveness of electrostatic inhalations in the treatment of such conditions as asthma. These may be administered as an electrostatic charge on fairly large water particles or by the use of air "ionizers". The charged ions produced by these instruments do not remain as single molecules sufficiently long to be inhaled as such but probably attract molecules of water vapour to form minute particles. It is certainly possible to administer a relatively large concentration of charged particles in this fashion but no controlled evidence that they are of any clinical value has been produced.

Inhaled Fibres

Asbestos fibres may be up to 200 or 300 μ long but have diameters of less than 1 μ. Fibres of similar shape are found in glass or viscose rayon factories. The aerodynamic properties of such particles were investigated by Timbrell (1965) who found that the terminal velocity of a fibre was virtually independent of its length but was approximately equal to that of a unit density sphere whose diameter was three times the diameter of the fibre.

He showed that such long fibres were able to penetrate to the alveoli because of their tendency to align themselves with their long axis parallel to the airflow. However, many are trapped by interception at the bifurcation of the small airways. Fibres of chrysotile asbestos are curved and probably have a greater tendency to be trapped before reaching the alveoli (Timbrell, 1970). This may be one reason why they do not appear to cause pleural mesotheliomas as do the straight fibres of crocidolite. Each type of asbestos mineral has several subgroups according to the geological conditions under which it was formed and the aerodynamic features of each play some part in its clinical affects. Crocidolite, for example, from some mines, is composed of relatively thick fibres having a high terminal velocity which may be unable to penetrate into the alveolar structure to the same degree as fine fibres from other mines and is associated with a correspondingly different pulmonary response (Timbrell *et al.*, 1971).

Physiological Protection against Dust

Coal seams contain thick bands composed almost entirely of vast quantities of pollen grains. These recall the time when wind dispersal was the only means of plant fertilization. The air in those days must have had even higher concentrations of organic matter than that of the present day. The first air breathing animals had to protect the gas exchange surfaces of their respiratory organs from this airborne dust and the requirement has continued ever since. The normal respiratory tract of man demonstrates the efficiency of the mechanisms which have evolved for this purpose.

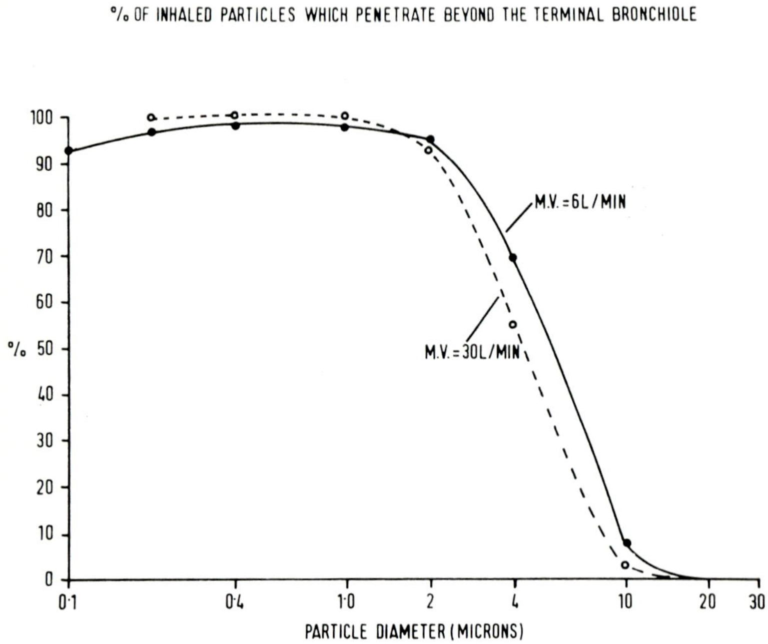

FIG. 4. Percentage of inhaled particles which are able to penetrate beyond the terminal bronchiole. Mouth breathing at rest and on moderate exercise. It is not implied that all such particles are deposited in the alveolus. Many are exhaled or trapped on the cilia during exhalation.

In this context the upper airways may be viewed as a protective filter which only allows certain fractions of inhaled dust to penetrate to the alveoli. The physiological efficiency of the filter is defined by the fraction of dust which is able to pass beyond the terminal bronchiole. This was calculated for the resting and exercising subject and the results are shown in Fig. 4. The curves are very similar and show that the "filter" is virtually independent of the rate of airflow. The explanation for this is that particle deposition is predominantly due to sedimentation at low rates of flow but due to impaction on exercise. The result is that no particle greater than about 20 μ is ever likely to reach the alveoli. This may be of physiological importance in that the macrophages themselves are about 20 μ in diameter and there is probably an upper limit to the size of particle which they can engulf. The special importance of fibrous particles may relate to their unique ability to reach the alveoli and yet to be too large to be removed by phagocytosis. The great cleansing power of macrophages for particles below this size is illustrated by the low concentrations of dust found in the lungs of coalminers despite the very great total dust burden deposited in them during a working lifetime.

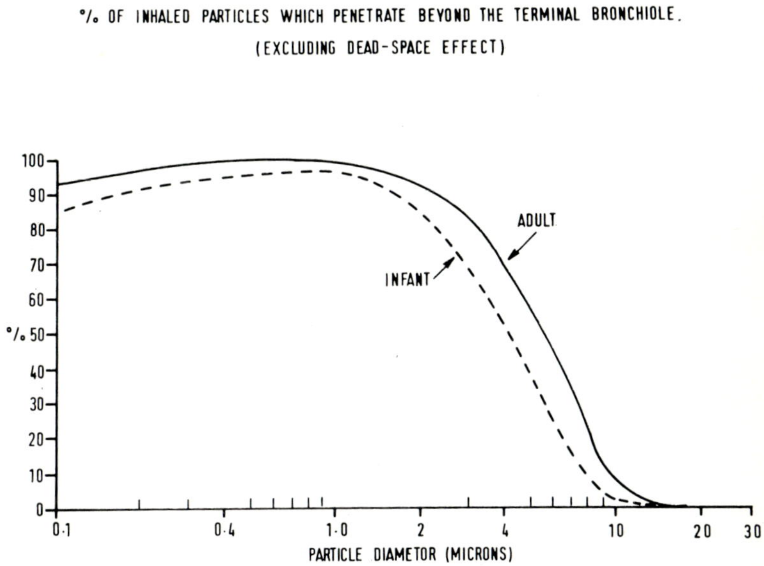

FIG. 5. Percentage of inhaled particles which are able to penetrate beyond the terminal bronchiole in the adult and in the infant. Mouth breathing at rest.

The small airways of children merit special consideration, not least because of the importance of aerosol therapy during childhood. The same calculations of the filtration efficiency of the ciliated airway illustrated in Fig. 5 were carried out from the newborn infant (Hislop *et al.*, 1971). The curve is very similar to that of the adult and suggests an equivalent protective action. The fine calibre of the airways of the infant might, at first, appear to form a more efficient filter for inhaled dust but the effect is surprisingly small.

Preventive Measures

Almost all of the airborne particulate matter causing disease of the lung is produced by man himself. The details of dust protection in industry are the province of the factory medical service or of the industrial hygienist. The aim must always be to reduce or remove the dust exposure if possible. This may sometimes be achieved by using alternative techniques such as the carborundum grinding wheel in place of sandstone, of shot blasting instead of sand blasting (the latter being now illegal in this country). If it is essential to employ a potentially dangerous process then special measures are required to reduce the amount of dust. Rock drills are thus provided with water feed mechanisms which damp the rock and reduce the airborne concentration of particles. Efficient exhaust ventilation is used to prevent the accumulation of dust at static working sites. If these precautions still leave undesirable amounts of dust in the air then workers must be protected by efficient mask respirators, and completely self contained air supplies must be provided for protection against the most dangerous dusts.

The use of respirators is never entirely satisfactory. The face pieces frequently do not fit and, if they are hot or uncomfortable, the workers will not use them. It should nevertheless be perfectly possible to make efficient use of respirators when the exposure is of short duration. Farmers unbaling mouldy hay, for example, are usually exposed to high concentrations of dust for brief periods only and protection during this time may be all that is necessary.

Major difficulties are encountered in recognizing that a hazard exists because there is often a long delay between the initial exposure and the appearance of disease. The same delay makes it difficult to define safety levels and to assess the results of their implication. The economic realities must also be considered. While, in theory, it is desirable to protect the whole population from any noxious dust whatsoever, this can never be achieved in an industrial society which must support a large population. It is, in fact, extremely difficult to show that general air pollution has any great effect on the individual and the single outstanding example of ill-health caused by airborne particles remains the cigarette.

References

Altshuler, B., Yarmus, L., Palmes, E. D. and Nelson, N. (1957), "Aerosol Deposition in the Human Respiratory Tract." *A.M.A. Arch. Ind. Health*, **15**, 293.

Altshuler, B. (1959), "Calculation of Regional Deposition of Aerosols in the Respiratory Tract." *Bull. Math. Biophys.*, **21**, 257.

Altshuler, B., Palmes, E. D. and Nelson, N. (1967), "Regional Aerosol Deposition in the Human Respiratory Tract." In *Inhaled Particles and Vapours II*, p. 323. Ed. C. N. Davies. London: Pergamon Press.

Arlidge, J. T. (1892), "The Hygiene Diseases and Mortality of Occupations," p. 249. London: Percival.

Bell, D. and Elmes, P. C. (1968), *Proc. 2nd Int. Cong. on the Biological Effects of Asbestos*. Dresden, 1968. In Press.

Beeckmans, J. M. (1965), "The Deposition of Aerosols in the Respiratory Tract." *Canad. J. Physiol. Pharm.*, **43**, 157.

Brain, J. D. (1971), "The Effects of Inhaled Particles on the Numbers of Alveolar Macrophages." In *Inhaled Particles* III, p. 209. Ed. W. H. Walton. London: Unwin.

Brown, C. E. (1931), "Quantitative Measurements of the Inhalation, Retention, and Exhalation of Dusts and Fumes by Man." *J. Ind. Hyg. Toxicol.*, **10,** 13.

Brown, J. H., Cook, K. M., Ney, F. G. and Hatch, T. (1950), "Influence of Particle Size upon the Retention of Particulate Matter in the Human Lung." *Am. J. Public Health*, **40,** 450.

Dautrebande, L., Beckmann, H. and Walkenhorst, W. (1957), "Lung Deposition of Fine Dust Particles." *A.M.A. Arch. Ind. Health*, **16,** 179.

Davies, C. N. (1964), "A Comparison between Inhaled Dust and the Dust Recovered from Human Lungs." *Health Physic*, **10,** 1029.

Davies, C. N. (1967), Editorial in *Inhaled Particles and Vapours* II, p. xiii. Ed. C. N. Davies. London: Pergamon Press.

Dennis, W. L. (1961), In *Inhaled Particles and Vapours*, p. 88. Ed. C. N. Davies. London: Pergamon Press.

Drinker, P., Thomson, R. M. and Finn, J. L. (1928), "Quantitative Measurements of the Inhalation, Retention and Exhalation of Dust and Fumes by Man." *J. Ind. Hyg. Toxicol.*, **10,** 13.

Einbrodt, H. J. (1967), "Experiments on the Elimination of Dust from Human Lungs." *Ann. Occup. Hyg.*, **10,** 47.

Findeisen, W. (1935), "Über das Absetzen Kleiner, in der Luft suspendierten Teilchen in der menschlichen Lunge bei der atmung." *Pflüger's Arch. ges. Physiol.*, **236,** 367.

Heppleston, A. G. (1961), "Observations on the Disposal of Inhaled Dust by Means of the Double Exposure Technique." In *Inhaled Particles and Vapours*, p. 320. Ed. C. N. Davies. London: Pergamon Press.

Heppleston, A. G. (1963), "The Disposal of Inhaled Particulate Matter; a Unifying Hypothesis." *Amer. J. Path.*, **42,** 119.

Hislop, A., Muir, D. C. F., Reid, L. McA., Jacobsen, M. and Simon, G. (1971), (Personal Communication).

Holma, B. (1967), "Lung Clearance of Mono- and Di-disperse Aerosols Determined by Profile Scanning and Whole-body Counting." *Acta Med. Scan.* Sup. No. 473.

Horsfield, K. and Cumming, G. (1968), "Functional Consequences of Airway Morphology." *J. Appl. Physiol.* **24,** 384.

Jacobsen, M., Rae, S., Walton, W. H. and Rogan, J. M. (1971), "The Relation between Pneumoconiosis and Dust Exposure in British Coal Mines." In *Inhaled Particles* III, p. 903. Ed. W. H. Walton. London: Unwin.

Klosterkotter, W. and Bunemann, G. (1961), "Animal Experiments on the Elimination of Inhaled Dust." In *Inhaled Particles and Vapours*, p. 372. Ed. C. N. Davies. London: Pergamon Press.

Landahl, H. D. and Herrmann, R. G. (1948), "On the Retention of Air-borne Particulates in the Human Lung." *J. Ind. Hyg. Toxicol.*, **30,** 181.

Landahl, H. D. (1950), "On the Removal of Air-borne Droplets by the Human Respiratory Tract. I. The Lung." *Bull. Math. Biophys.*, **12,** 43.

Landahl, H. D., Tracewell, T. N. and Lassen, W. H. (1952), "Retention of Air-borne Particulates in the Human Lung." *A.M.A. Arch. Ind. Hyg. Occ. Med.*, **6,** 508.

Le Bouffant, L. (1961), "Etude Quantitative de L'epuration Pulmonaire chez Le Rat; Comparaison Entre Poussières Inertes et Poussières Nocives." In *Inhaled Particles and Vapours*, p. 369. Ed. C. N. Davies. London: Pergamon Press.

Lehmann, G. (1935), "Dust Filtering Efficiency of the Human Nose and its Significance in the Causation of Silicosis." *J. Ind. Hyg.*, **17,** 37.

Lippman, M. and Albert, R. E. (1969), "The Effect of Particle Size on the Regional Deposition of Inhaled Aerosols in the Human Respiratory Tract." *Amer. Ind. Hyg. Ass. J.*, **30,** 257.

Lippman, M., Albert, R. E. and Peterson, H. T. (1971), "The Regional Deposition of Inhaled Aerosols in Man." In *Inhaled Particles* III, p. 105. Ed. W. H. Walton. London: Unwin.

Lister, J. (1868), "An Address on the Antiseptic System of Treatment in Surgery." *Brit. Med. J.*, **2,** 53.

Love, R. G., Muir, D. C. F. and Sweetland, K. F. (1971), "Aerosol Deposition in the Lungs of Coalworkers." In *Inhaled Particles* III, p. 131. Ed. W. H. Walton. London: Unwin.

McRae, J. (1913), *The Ash of Silicotic Lungs.* Johannesburg: South African Institute for Medical Research.

Muir, D. C. F. and Davies, C. N. (1967), "The Deposition of 0·5 micron Diameter Aerosols in the Lungs of Man." *Ann. Occup. Hyg.*, **10,** 161.

Owens, J. S. (1923). "Dust in Expired Air." *Trans. Med. Soc.* (*Lond.*), **45,** 79.

Proctor, D. F., Swift, D. L., Quinlan, M., Salmon, S., Takagi, Y. and Evering, S. (1969), "The Nose and Man's Atmospheric Environment." *A.M.A. Arch. Envir. Hlth.*, **18,** 671.

Proctor, D. F. and Swift, D. L. (1971), "The Nose—a Defence Against the Atmospheric Environment." In *Inhaled Particles* III, p. 59. Ed. W. H. Walton. London: Unwin.

Sanchis, J., Dolovitch, M., Chalmers, R. and Newhouse, M. (1971), "Regional Distribution and Lung Clearance Mechanisms in Smokers and Non-smokers." In *Inhaled Particles* III, p. 183. Ed. W. H. Walton. London: Unwin.

Schiller, E. (1961), "Inhalation, Retention and Elimination of Dusts from Dogs' and Rats' Lungs with Special Reference to the Alveolar Phagocytes and Bronchial Apithelium." In *Inhaled Particles* II, p. 342. Ed. C. N. Davies. London: Pergamon Press.

Stöber, W., Einbrodt, H. J. and Klosterkötter, W. (1967), "Quantitative Studies of Dust Retention in Animal and Human Lungs after Chronic Inhalation." In *Inhaled Particles and Vapours* II, p. 409. Ed. C. N. Davies. London: Pergamon Press.

Thomson, M. L. and Short, M. D. (1969), "Mucociliary Function in Health, Chronic Obstructive Airway Disease, and Asbestosis." *J. Appl. Physiol.*, **26,** 535.

Timbrell, V. (1965), "The Inhalation of Fibrous Dusts." *Ann. New York Acad. Sci.*, **132,** 255.

Timbrell, V. (1970), "The Inhalation of Fibres." In Pneumoconiosis, p. 3. Ed. Shapiro, Oxford: Oxford University Press.

Timbrell, V., Griffiths, D.M. and Pooley, F. D. (1971), "Possible Biological Importance of Fibre Diameters of South African Amphiboles." *Nature*, **232,** 55.

Tyndall, J. (1870), "On Dust and Disease." *Proc. Roy. Inst.*, **6,** 1.

Van Wijk, A. M. and Patterson, H. S. (1940), "The Percentage of Particles of Different Sizes Removed from Dust-laden Air by Breathing." *J. Ind. Hyg. Toxicol.*, **22,** 31.

West, J. B. (1965), *Ventilation/blood flow and gas exchange.* Oxford: Blackwell Scientific Publications.

Wright, B. M. (1961), Discussion in *Inhaled Particles and Vapours*, p. 398. Ed. C. N. Davies. London: Pergamon Press.

Chapter 2

Air Pollution and Tobacco Smoke

P. J. LAWTHER

There are special difficulties to be met in attempting to write a chapter on air pollution and tobacco smoke in a book on aerosols: the limitations of space obviously preclude the presentation of anything more than an outline of the subject; particulate pollution cannot be considered properly in isolation from the gases which almost invariably accompany it, and most people these days are exposed to both air pollution and tobacco smoke which makes the distinction between their separate effects difficult and, in many cases, impossible. Likewise the changes in pollution and the increase in the habit of tobacco smoking makes difficult the assessment of the roles they play in the production of chronic disease. Yet a further complication is the great complexity of the physical nature and chemical composition of air pollution and tobacco smoke. Against these difficulties must be set the advantage of having the opportunity to discuss air pollution in conjunction with tobacco smoke, for all too often the effects on health of these two noxious aerosols are discussed as if they were separate subjects, whereas it is wiser to regard tobacco smoking as an assault on the body by an intense concentration of a special pollutant.

Air pollution and smoking have rightly been the subjects of intensive investigation and there is now an enormous amount (which is rapidly increasing) of published work of greatly varied quality; a critical review of the literature cannot be undertaken in a chapter which must needs be but an outline of the problem and to facilitate further study a list is appended of selected monographs, bibliographies, reviews and current abstracts to which reference should be made. In this essay an attempt will be made to add a sense of perspective to two environmental factors which are menacing the health of the public, and to remove some popular misconceptions which commonly cause confusion to the non-specialist.

Common Sources of Pollution

Aerosols derived from vegetation, "natural" processes such as volcanic eruptions, and industry have been discussed elsewhere. The commonest source of man-made pollution is the combustion of fuel for the generation of power, heat and transport. When pure hydrocarbon fuels are burned completely no aerosols are produced but when they are contaminated by sulphur compounds, halogen-containing substances and inorganic matter, fine particles may be produced even when combustion is efficient. Coal, oil or gas containing sulphur will produce oxides of which about 95% may be emitted as SO_2 and 5% as SO_3 or H_2SO_4 (the proportions emitted as the higher oxide or acid will depend in part on the temperature of burning); the sulphur trioxide will eventually absorb water to form droplets of sulphuric acid the size of which will depend on the initial acid content and the ambient humidity, and the sulphur dioxide is usually oxidized at rates which depend on concentration, the presence of water droplets and dissolved catalysts, to form sulphuric acid and sulphate (principally ammonium). When coal is burned much of the sulphur it contains may be retained in inorganic form in the ash. These droplets may grow sufficiently to fall as acid rain. Oxides of nitrogen which may subsequently form droplets of nitric acid are formed by fixation of atmospheric nitrogen and from nitrogen in fuel. Hydrochloric and hydrofluoric acids are emitted from some fuels but ambient concentrations high enough to affect human health have not been found. Fine ash may be emitted after being carried up the flues by draught and large industrial power plants are usually fitted with grit arrestors to prevent emission of such particles. More usually ash is emitted as particles which are coarse enough to fall out near to their source and, because of their comparatively large size, cannot penetrate far into the lung and therefore are a nuisance rather than a hazard to health.

By far the commonest particulate pollutant at breathing level is the smoke which is derived from inadequate combustion of coal and, less frequently, oil. If a simple hydrocarbon is burnt in an inadequate supply of air, fine particles, usually aggregated lamp black or polymers of high carbon content, are produced (Fig. 1). When coal is burned inefficiently, as is so often the case (in the British open coal fire the smokeless combustion of bituminous coal is impossible), large quantities of tarry droplets are produced in addition to particles of soot. These particles which are produced largely by distillation may contain very many organic compounds, including phenols, bases, acids and hydrocarbons, of which the most notorious are the polycyclic aromatic hydrocarbons, some of which are carcinogenic. These compounds have been studied widely because of their relevance to the problem of the causation of human lung cancer; moreover Commins (1969) has shown that the ratios of the concentrations of certain hydrocarbons to each other in air is so critically dependent on the fuel to air ratio during their formation that these ratios may be used to determine the relative contributions made by coal fires and motor vehicles. Many trace elements may be emitted from fossil fuels and the relevance of these pollutants to human health is being studied by many workers.

Motor vehicles as sources of pollution merit separate mention: they produce localized low-level pollution by particles and gases and that

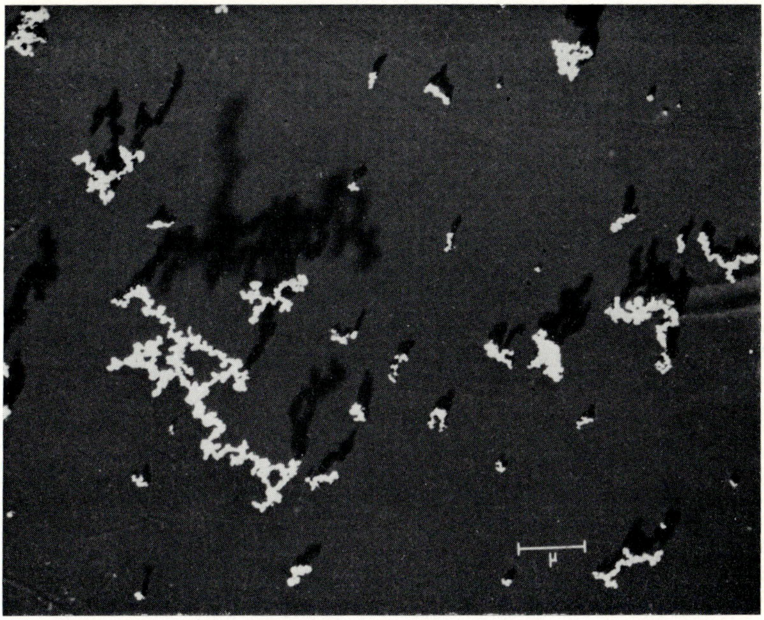

FIG. 1. Smoke aggregates found in urban air shadowed with gold-palladium. Negative print.

emitted by petrol engines differs in many respects from the exhaust products of diesel engines. Petrol engines (spark ignition) burn fuel in an essentially "rich" mixture so that commonly hydrocarbons and carbon monoxide are emitted in considerable quantities—in the diesel engine (compression ignition) fuel is burnt in a large excess of air and the emission of hydrocarbons and carbon monoxide is usually negligible. The petrol engine emits lead, usually as halide, derived from tetra-ethyl or tri-methyl lead added as anti-detonants to prevent "pinking".

Robinson and Ludwig (1967) have studied the size of the lead particles emitted in three cities in the USA and reported that 75% of the mass was less than 0·42 μ diameter. They found up to 9 $\mu g/m^3$ in Los Angeles. The concentration in a busy street in London (measured over a year) was 3·2 $\mu g/m^3$ compared with a "background" level (measured in the city but away from the street) of 0·8 $\mu g/m^3$ (Waller, Commins and Lawther, 1965).

Diesel engines emit no lead but both types of engine may emit varying quantities of burnt or unburnt lubricating oils which may contain metallic additives such as barium. The diesel engine can produce spectacular and disgusting amounts of black smoke if it is maladjusted, worn or overloaded. When starting from cold, aerosols of unburnt fuel

Table 1

Common polycyclic hydrocarbons in smoke

Hydrocarbon	*Carcinogenicity*	*Hydrocarbon*	*Carcinogenicity*
Naphthalene	−	3,4-benzfluoranthene	+
Acenaphthylene	−	10,11-benzfluoranthene	+++
Fluorene	−	11,12-benzfluoranthene	−
Anthracene	−	Perylene	−
Phenanthrene	−	1,2-benzpyrene	+
Pyrene	−	3,4-benzpyrene	+++
Fluoranthene	−	1,12-benzperylene	−
1,2-benzfluorene	−	Anthanthrene	−
3,4-benzfluorene	−	2,3(o-phenylene)pyrene	+
1,2-benzanthracene	+	Coronene	−
Chrysene	+		

may be emitted and these can be intensely irritant to the eyes and respiratory tract. The smoke, accompanied by carbon monoxide, is usually almost pure carbon and contains polycyclic hydrocarbons in amounts which are very small in comparison with those found in coal smoke. Among the many complex organic compounds emitted by both types of engine are those which give the exhausts their characteristic smell. Petrol contains negligible amounts of sulphur and diesel fuel, while containing about 0·4% sulphur, produces negligible quantities of SO_2. It is important to mention the fact that certain hydrocarbons, notably olefines emitted in petrol exhausts can in the presence of oxides of nitrogen and strong sunlight take part in complex photochemical reactions with the production of the lachrymatory haze known as "Los Angeles smog".

Industrial processes may pollute the air with an understandably wide variety of substances some of which, like beryllium and asbestos, have produced disease among the general public. Other pollutants from industry such as iron oxide fume and cement dust produce serious annoyance rather than disease. In Britain, industrial emissions are kept under close surveillance by the Alkali Inspectorate.

Having discussed briefly the main sources of urban air pollution there is a need to emphasize strongly the need to distinguish between emissions and ground level concentrations. All too frequently confusion is caused by disproportionate attention being paid to figures of dramatic magnitude relating to the amounts of pollutant emitted when what matters to the clinician is the concentration and amount at lung level which may be inhaled. Again, in this context, motor vehicles need special mention since in most places they produce pollution which is surprisingly limited in extent, the concentrations of exhaust products falling away very rapidly as the distance from the road increases.

Notable exceptions are places such as Los Angeles in which the emissions from many vehicles accumulate in large masses of stagnant air and are involved in complex photo-chemical reactions.

Distribution of air pollutants and the relationship between emissions and concentrations at lung level will depend on many factors which must be considered carefully when sampling sites are being selected. Height of source and velocity of emission; exposure of the surrounding terrain; the presence of nearby buildings and the weather and climate all play an important part in determining the degree of dispersion. There is no doubt that the most serious contribution to pollution at ground level in many countries is made by the inefficient combustion of domestic fuels, the products of which are discharged near the ground. The most dangerous weather is that when temperature inversions cause stagnation and consequently fumigation.

Sampling Methods and Measurement

Sampling methods and sites will be selected according to the needs of the survey or experiment. A convenient critical review of commonly used methods has been written by Ellison (1965) whose adjacent article (1965) "The Particles in Town Air" is an excellent account of the subject. Selection of sites and methods of sampling in towns may be based on several principles: the town may be divided into areas by a geometric grid each area of which contains a fixed sampler, or a sampler may be moved on a strictly random basis from one grid space to another at predetermined intervals. For other purposes a town may be divided into different areas based on the activity of the population—residential, commercial or industrial—with fixed samplers at the "centre of gravity" of population in each area. Similarly selected areas of residential, commercial or industrial districts may be used as sites for fixed samplers. Finally, members of population to be studied may be selected at random and fitted with "personal" samplers; in some cases, where the particulate pollutant is absorbed, as in the case of lead, analyses of blood or urine samples of members of the population are greatly to be preferred to those of air samples as they indicate true exposure and body burden. The use of certain out-moded methods must be avoided because they may give misleading results: air pollution used to be measured by collecting deposited matter but it should be realized that comparatively coarse matter collected in deposit gauges is that which causes annoyance rather than disease. Likewise, the use of the lead peroxide candle to measure SO_2 has been discontinued, not because it did not measure the degree of sulphation for which it was designed (to assess damage to buildings), but because the supposed SO_2 figures it gave were not appropriate for use in epidemiological research.

These methods of assessing solid matter and SO_2 have been replaced by the use of the DSIR "volumetric" samplers in which air is filtered through a Whatman No. 1 filter paper on which the smoke (or "black suspended matter") leaves a stain, the reflectance of which can be related by reference to a calibration curve to the weight of smoke in the air. After filtration the air is bubbled through dilute peroxide solution in which SO_2 is oxidized to the more easily titratable sulphuric acid (titration is done to pH 4·5 to avoid interference by atmospheric CO_2). Suspended matter varies in blackness and calibrations of stains in gravimetric terms must be reviewed as pollutions change. Net acidity (acids, usually sulphuric minus base), may be determined by titration of the filter papers. This "volumetric" method of assessment of pollution is widely used and the results of measurements made in many towns in Great Britain are collated by the Department of Trade and Industry at Warren Spring Laboratory and published. These data are very useful in epidemiological work in coalburning countries. But this apparatus gives results which describe pollution only in terms of "total black suspended matter" and sulphur dioxide, and obviously other more elaborate and specific methods are needed to supplement these for purposes of research.

Larger samples to be used for chemical analysis of particulate pollutants may be obtained from "high volume" samplers in which air is drawn by means of a vacuum cleaner motor through a glass fibre filter "paper". (These glass fibre filters have much lower resistance to air flow than paper filters; the glass from which the fibres are spun is slightly alkaline and this property precludes the use of these filters for the collection of samples for determination of acid by titration.) Flow rates of approximately 1·5 m^3/min. are usually used and permit the collection of samples for analysis over relatively short periods of time: samples may be weighed directly. Table 2 gives a list of substances (including gases) found in the air of London with their highest hourly concentrations observed since 1954.

The cascade impactor originally described by May (1945) may be used to enable the size distribution of airborne particles to be assessed. Air is aspirated through a series of jets of diminishing size and the apparatus is so designed that each stage is a more efficient collector of particles than the preceding one. Particles are collected on glass slides for examination by microscope. The finest particles may be collected on a filter which is added as a fifth stage. Properties other than particle size may be examined by modifying the glass slides on which the particles are collected and Waller (1963) has used gelatine coated thymol blue impregnated slides to study the acid particles often present in town air.

The thermal precipitator (described by Green and Lane, 1957) collects particles by thermophoresis and despite the slow rate of sampling has many advantages, chief among which is its efficiency for collection of small particles for examination under the light or electron microscopes. By the use of the cascade impactor and thermal precipitator much has

Table 2

Some pollutants found in the air of the City of London
(Arranged in descending order of highest concentrations observed since 1954)

Pollutant	*Highest hourly concentration* ($\mu g/m^3$ *air*)
Carbon dioxide	2,520,000
Carbon monoxide	68,700*
Particulate matter (smoke)	9,700
Sulphur dioxide	5,650
Nitric oxide	1,350
Sulphate (water soluble)	666
Sulphuric acid	680
Nitrogen dioxide	470
Chloride (water soluble)	410
Calcium	82
Hydrogen sulphide	70
Ammonia (gas)	56
Sodium	33
Iron	25
Zinc	24
Lead	22
Nitrate	5
Manganese	5
Chromium	2
Vanadium	2
Copper	2
Tin	2
3,4-benzpyrene	2
Nickel	1
Cadmium	1
Titanium	1
Molybdenum, cobalt, bismuth, antimony, beryllium, barium	<1

* Street sample

been learned about the chemical and physical nature of particles found in town air; Table 3 shows some estimates of size, number and mass concentration in samples taken in different conditions in London. Because the particles vary widely in composition and shape it is impossible to give precise assessments of size but the mass median diameter can be said to be generally less than 1 μm.

The electron microscope is therefore of obvious value in the study of the nature of particulate pollution and has been used to good effect by Waller, Brooks and Cartwright (1963); Waller and Biles (1964) and Horstman and Wagman (1967).

Obviously the time taken to collect samples must depend on the

Table 3

Number and size of particles in London air

Sampling site	*No. of particles/ml*	*No. median diameter* (μm)	*Estimated conc.* ($\mu g/m^3$)	*Mass median diameter* (μm)
City, normal pollution	7,800	0·09	100	0·7
City, moderate pollution	27,100	0·09	370	0·8
City, high pollution	154,500	0·10	1,970	0·9
Street sample, light traffic	27,300	0·12	280	0·5
Tunnel sample, heavy traffic	120,400	0·09	1,260	0·7

reason for collection. Concentrations may vary by a factor of 20 within short periods and for the study of acute immediate effects continuous monitoring or the collection of hourly samples may be needed. For the study of long-term effects and for the assessment of trends in pollution in relation to mortality and morbidity samples taken over 24 hour periods or longer, or means of daily concentrations, may suffice.

Again it must be emphasized that sampling techniques and sites must be chosen with great care and results obtained therefrom interpreted with caution. Urban air contains many compounds which may react together in the atmosphere, on filters, in bubblers or even in the lung. Some are unstable; some particles have adsorbed gases and liquids on their surfaces; some are decomposed by light or air either on filters or in solution in the laboratory after collection. Rarely are the methods used for their analysis and determination wholly specific or free from interference by other substances. Careful reference should be made to the literature and especially to WHO or OECD monographs in order to select the methods appropriate to the proposed study. Especially in epidemiological research the site from which samples are taken is of great importance, and much can be learned by studying the methods employed by the Department of Trade and Industry (Warren Spring Laboratory) in their National Survey which is described in the 32nd Report on the Investigation of Atmospheric Pollution (1967); Waller's essay (1966) on "The interpretation and use of data on air pollution in epidemiological research" is a useful guide.

Tobacco Smoke

The smoke from burning tobacco smoke is a complex mixture of gases, liquid droplets and uncondensed compounds and as it is inhaled it contains many millions of particles per ml. The mean median diameter has been reported (Harris, 1960) as 0·16 μm and 0·5 μm by Albert and Nelson (1964) but the size of the droplets will depend, among other factors, on the ambient humidity. Fig. 2 shows an electron micrograph of cigarette smoke aerosol collected in the free air.

The physical properties of tobacco smoke as determined in the ambient air are of limited relevance to the penetration of, and retention in, the respiratory tract since their hygroscopicity renders them subject to changes in size on inhalation.

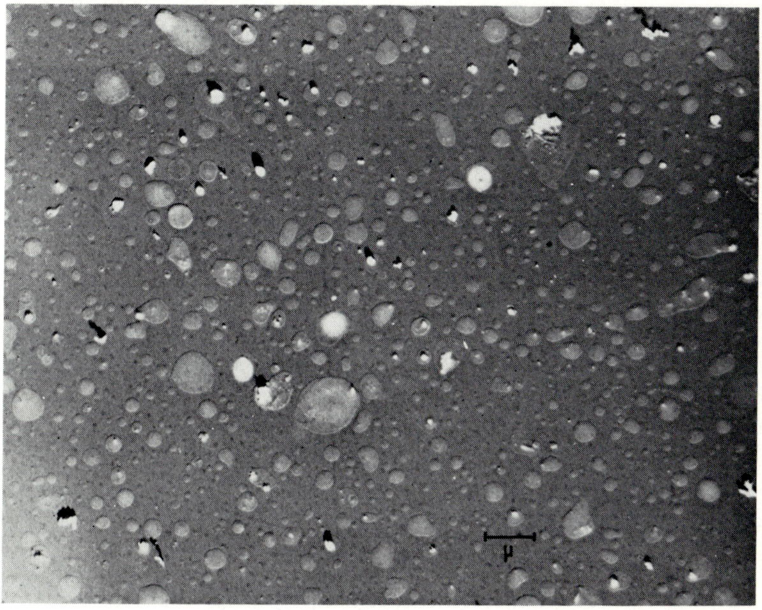

FIG. 2. Appearance of droplets from cigarette smoke aerosol. Shadowed with gold-palladium. Negative print.

The chemical nature of particles of tobacco smoke is very complex indeed and varies with type of tobacco, whether it is smoked in cigarettes, pipes or cigars, the manner of smoking, whether it is sampled as side stream or main stream smoke (i.e. whether it is taken as it enters the atmosphere from the site of incineration or as it would enter the mouth).

Its chemistry is too complex to be discussed in detail here and the reader is referred especially to the excellent report "Smoking and Health" (1964, U.S. Department of Health, Education and Welfare; Public Health Service), and the supplementary reviews (1967 and 1968) entitled "The Health Consequences of Smoking". These publications are notable especially for the bibliographies. Of equal value are the periodic publications of the (British) Tobacco Research Council. The Reports of the Royal College of Physicians "Smoking and Health" (1962, 1971), two of the most important works concerning the effect of any factor on the public health are paramount in their assessment of the problem in the UK but less complete in discussion of the chemical and physical nature of the pollutant.

The particulate phase of tobacco smoke contains very many compounds among which are aliphatic, alicydic, polycyclic and isoprenoid hydrocarbons, alcohols, phenols, acids, aldehydes, acetones, steroids, amino acids and alkaloids. The tar is carcinogenic to mouse skin, co-carcinogenic (mainly by virtue of its phenolic content) and, of course, the pharmacologically active constituent to which many become addicted in the true sense, is nicotine.

Prominent among the gaseous constituents (which cannot be ignored when discussing the aerosol component) are carbon monoxide and nitric oxide.

Tobacco smoke must be considered both as a pollutant inhaled in very high concentrations by smokers, and as an "aged" aerosol which can contaminate the ambient air and act as an irritant to smoker and non-smoker. There is good evidence that smoke undergoes changes, both physical and chemical, after liberation into the ambient air from either side stream or after exhalation.

The differences in the chemical nature of smokes from cigarettes, pipes and cigars already mentioned are many and great and, because of the observed different effects on health, are the subject of intense study.

The Effects of Polluted Air on Health

There is no doubt that when pollution in towns exceeds certain levels associated increases in mortality and morbidity may be clearly demonstrated. The closeness of the association depends mainly on the severity of the pollution and the frailty of those subjected to it. The agents responsible for these effects have not yet been identified with any degree of certainty, despite an immense amount of work both experimental and by the use of epidemiological techniques. A different problem, more difficult to solve and of great importance, is the assessment of the part played by pollution in the causation of disease. Among the difficulties encountered in attempts to solve both of these problems are the facts that particulate pollution is always associated with gaseous pollutants; that pollutants are rarely present in concentrations high enough to lead one to expect positive results from laboratory experiments on normal subjects (one cannot justify on ethical grounds experimental exposure of persons with respiratory disease who are known to be susceptible to the harmful effects of urban pollution to anything more than minute concentrations of simplest suspect substances); that the diseases in which pollution is thought to play a part (principally chronic bronchitis and lung cancer) are multifactorial, take a long time to develop, or are apparently inextricably linked to smoking.

The effect of air pollution on man is most easily seen when contaminants accumulate and reach high concentrations in towns during the winter when anti-cyclonic conditions lead to temperature inversions and stagnation of the air. Radiation fogs frequently accompany the pollutants in these conditions and make even more complex the chemistry and physics of the contaminating gases and particles. In the notorious London "smog" of December 1952 there was an increase in mortality which has been assessed as being equivalent to over 4,000 deaths in the week of the fog. More deaths attributable to the pollution would have occurred later and were not manifest as a peak in the mortality curves. There is evidence that these acute episodes of high pollution are associated with increases in morbidity and that some patients attribute, with good reason, the onset of serious symptoms of bronchitis or heart failure to peaks in pollution. It is possible that repeated exposure to high levels of pollution may be a factor in the development of chronic bronchitis.

The changes in morbidity and mortality in the London (1952) episode have been described and discussed in detail (Ministry of Health, 1954). Not surprisingly, the "excess" deaths occurred among those sections of the population least able to cope with added stress: the elderly, the very young, and those suffering already from diseases of the respiratory and cardio-vascular systems. There was also seen an increase in deaths from coronary artery disease and cerebrovascular accidents. Two urgent tasks confronted those concerned with the health of the public: to identify the pollutant or mixture of pollutants responsible for the deaths, the exacerbation of existing illness and the breakdown in health, and to protect the susceptible people against the bad effects of subsequent episodes by the prohibition of the emission of the offending pollutants or as an iterim measure, by the provision of such protective devices as masks and "air conditioners".

To approach these tasks rationally it was necessary to consider the clinical picture and the mechanisms by which the observed disturbances were produced. Clinical evidence of increase in airway resistance produced by bronchospasm or hypersecretion of mucus, or by both, was easily obtained, and subsequent research on the acute effects of high levels of air pollution has been concentrated on the need to identify contaminants capable of causing irritation of the bronchial tree when exhibited in concentrations similar to those encountered in "smogs".

Sulphur dioxide is an irritant gas when inhaled in relatively high concentrations and it is capable of evoking bronchospasm and the hypersecretion of mucus. Despite the paucity of reliable estimates of the concentration of this gas during the 1952 episode it is reasonable, in the light of measurements made then and during subsequent incidents when pollution has been high, to assume that it is unlikely to have exceeded 2 ppm. Much experimental work on animals and on normal subjects has been done and there is little reliable evidence that this gas, by itself, could have caused the effects observed.

Particulate matter, in all its complexity discussed briefly above, was obviously suspect. There is evidence that particulate matter which is chemically relatively inert (such as carbon black, indian ink aerosols, aluminium powder, etc.) can cause increases in airway resistance if inhaled in high enough concentrations but coal smoke, fresh or aged in the atmosphere, is more likely to be active in this respect, if indeed it is proved to be active, by virtue of its chemical constitution rather than by its mere physical form.

Among the particles found in polluted air sulphuric acid is rightly suspected of having irritant properties and the possibility that sulphur dioxide may be adsorbed on carbon particles has lead to the search for evidence of synergistic effects of gaseous and particulate pollutants. Many methods have been used in this field: much of the experimental work using animals is irrelevant because of the high concentrations used and on the rare occasions when positive findings have been obtained when realistic amounts have been inhaled, repetition of the experiments on human volunteers has produced negative results.

The failure, as yet, to identify, with any degree of certainty of the pollutant or combination of pollutants responsible for the clinical picture seen to be associated with exposure to high levels of pollution may be due to several reasons: the compounds selected for experimental inhalation are usually relatively simple substances known to be irritant in high concentrations; the active substance may yet be shown to be some complex organic chemical capable of producing bronchospasm in its own right or by provoking the release of histamine or some allied substance. It is likewise possible that the need, on ethical grounds, to use only healthy volunteers as subjects for experimental inhalations has misled many investigators; increases in airway resistance so small as to be hard to discern even by the use of the whole body plethysmograph are tolerated without any disturbance by the normal subject but may yet have serious consequences if they lead to gross disturbances in ventilation/perfusion relationships in non-homogenous lungs, by which serious degrees of arterial desaturation may be produced. The methods most commonly used to estimate airway resistance or changes in ventilatory capacity have disadvantages in that most of them require some artificial manoeuvre which, in itself, can produce increases or decreases in resistance. The maximum expiratory effort required in the measurement of the timed forced expiratory volume and the peak expiratory flow rate can produce artefactual changes which may obscure changes which might have been produced by the experimental inhalation. In the use of the whole body plethysmograph to determine respiratory resistance the subject is required to pant against a closed shutter and this unnatural procedure may produce changes unrelated to the inhalation of the suspect pollutant.

There is obviously a good case for the development of techniques for examining changes in lung function during normal breathing. The examination of respiratory flow patterns measured at length at rest has obvious advantages and can be used to study the effect on patients of "natural" variations in pollution, though the decline in air pollution in England, to be discussed later, makes such studies more difficult than they would have formerly been when episodes of high pollution occurred only too frequently.

There remains the very real possibility that "acute" pollution acts, not solely by causing an increase in resistance to air flow within the respiratory tract but by interfering with the mechanical properties of the lung in some other way which would increase the work of breathing or otherwise impair lung function. If, for example, inhaled particles were to interfere with alveolar surfactant or its regeneration the consequent decrease, regional or total, in lung compliance may have serious effects on a lung already damaged by disease.

The search to identify the guilty pollutant continues and the use of new methods for the assessment of changes in lung function is welcome.

A considerable advantage of the Wright Peak Flow Meter is that it affords a simple means of assessing ventilatory function which can be used by many people with little training. This method is especially useful for use outside the laboratory for the study of the reactions of patients and normal subjects to daily variations in pollution. The meter can be loaned to bronchitic patients for their own daily assessment of ventilatory capacity so that it may be correlated with daily changes in pollution. This technique has already given promising results in some hands.

The epidemiological approach to the study of variations of pollution in relation to health is both complementary and supplementary to the use of the experimental method. In its crudest form, gross variations in pollution are seen to be associated with relatively gross variations in mortality if the populations studied are large enough.

Smaller variations between pollution and mortality and morbidity may be seen if the indices are chosen carefully and the populations studied are large enough. It must not be forgotten that the response of a population to the stress imposed by pollution is dependent not merely on the intensity of the pollution but also on the degree of susceptibility of the population; for healthy people will not die, nor be made acutely ill by lesser increases in pollution. This fact makes more attractive the use of patients with severe disease of the respiratory or cardiac systems in studying the effects of variations in pollution. Patients who attend chest clinics have been used to good effect by seeking their co-operation in reporting daily the variations they feel in the state of their health and by plotting these reports against pollution. It has been shown (Lawther, Waller and Henderson, 1970) that even minor changes in pollution as indicated by measurement of smoke and sulphur dioxide are closely related to daily changes in subjective assessments of well-being of patients.

So far only the effect of pollution as a cause of exacerbating existing disease has been discussed. The evidence from current research would tend to incriminate particulate rather than gaseous pollutants though the possibility remains that such gases as sulphur dioxide might be active when adsorbed on particles. The assessment of the part played by pollution in causing chronic lung disease, rather than in aggravating it, is important.

There are two main phases in the development of the florid clinical picture of advanced chronic bronchitis which all too often is accompanied by the development of emphysema. In simple chronic bronchitis, clinically manifest by chronic cough and the expectoration of mucoid sputum, the essential lesion is hypertrophy of the mucus secreting tissue of the respiratory tract generally in response to the irritation caused by the inhalation of cigarette smoke. Some airways obstruction is inevitable since the hypertrophic mucosa and its secretion decreases the calibre of the airways. There are good reasons, derived from results from experimental work and epidemiological studies, that if smoking ceases, these changes regress. But frequently simple chronic bronchitis is followed by infection of the lung; at first the infection is episodic and gives more to sporadic fibrile episodes; later the infection becomes chronic and leads to destruction of the lung parenchyma. Air pollution may play an important part in this second, more serious phase, of chronic bronchitis.

The study of the evolution of chronic bronchitis is made difficult by the fact that its natural history is long. In recent years the value of studying children, from birth and thereafter on a cohort basis, has been recognized and in some investigations, among which is that of Douglas and Waller (1966), the effect of pollution in favouring the development of lower respiratory infection even in infancy has been convincingly demonstrated.

The commonly held belief that the pollutant responsible for the development of chronic bronchitis is a simple chemical irritant such as sulphur dioxide or sulphuric acid may be doubted since the concentration of these substances commonly found in town air is so much lower than those commonly found in industrial atmospheres in which, despite the presumed irritation there is not a proportionate excess in the prevalence of chronic bronchitis.

The sputum of patients with infective chronic bronchitis commonly contains Haemophilus influenzae though its role as the predominant pathogen is disputed. A finding which may have some bearing on the development of the disease is that the growth of this organism is apparently stimulated *in vitro* by the presence of particulate matter, predominantly coal smoke (Lawther, Emerson and O'Grady, 1969). More recently there would seem to be some evidence that this apparent stimulation is due to the inhibition of the common form of the organism which allows the overgrowth of a phenotypically different strain. Whilst the relevance of this finding may be limited it could serve to stress the fact that pollution might play a more complex part in the cause of the disease than by virtue of its mere chemical irritancy.

The same effect on Haemophilus influenzae can be seen when cigarette tar is added to the culture. The role of cigarette smoking in the development of chronic bronchitis has been amply demonstrated in many investigations (Royal College of Physicians, 1971) though this mechanism by which it produces its effect may yet need further elucidation. There is no doubt that cigarette smoke is irritant, can cause bronchospasm, can inhibit ciliary activity and provokes secretion of mucus. This interference with bronchial clearance may be critical.

The presence of carcinogenic hydrocarbons in the particulate phase of town air pollution has already been mentioned briefly. Lung cancer is found more commonly in towns than in country areas, and the assumption, on superficial consideration of the problem, that the cause of lung cancer is coal smoke would appear to be justified. There is no doubt that such polycyclic hydrocarbons as 3:4 benzpyrene can be carcinogenic to man as well as to the skin of experimental animals. It is likely that the cancer of the scrotum in chimney sweeps described by Percivall Pott in 1775, mule spinners' cancer, and pitch workers' cancer were all due to this or allied compounds. The comparatively small excess of lung cancer seen among retort house workers in gas works in the air of which there was a vast excess of polycyclic hydrocarbons, may have been due to 3:4 benzpyrene. But it is wholly unreasonable to attribute the modern epidemic of lung cancer to air pollution by coal smoke since this disease has been rising alarmingly at the same time as pollution from coal smoke has been declining at an almost equally spectacular rate.

At one time some thought that the motor vehicle, especially the diesel engine, the exhaust of which is all too often visible because the engine is maladjusted or overloaded, was the cause of the recent rise in lung cancer but happily this is not so. There can be no doubt that the overwhelmingly major cause of the disease is cigarette smoking and the reader is referred to the Royal College of Physicians' Report "Smoking and Health Today" (1971) for a lucid exposition of contemporary evidence.

Sadly, the case against cigarette smoking is all too often based only on its association with lung cancer. Its relationship to chronic bronchitis has been mentioned briefly but in addition the habit plays a major part in the production of cardio-vascular disease. It is probable that carbon monoxide, in addition to the nicotine present in the droplet phase, plays a significant part in this process.

Whilst there would seem to be excellent reasons to encourage the search for a safer cigarette and in the meantime to encourage the cigarette smoker who cannot eschew tobacco to change to pipe smoking or to cigars, there are dangers in both these counsels. The development of a safer cigarette may well be based on the need to reduce the tar content of the smoke since there is adequate proof that the tar from cigarette condensate is carcinogenic, albeit weakly, to animal skin. The tar phase contains the nicotine to which many smokers are addicted. If one postulates that the addict will smoke to absorb a standard dose to which he has been accustomed and that the carcinogen, or co-carcinogen is in the gas phase rather than in the tar then the safer cigarette may yet be a more dangerous one. The carbon monoxide will, presumably remain since combustion will remain virtually unaltered. And it may take 25 years before we know whether the safer cigarette is indeed safer or more dangerous.

There is clearly less risk of getting lung cancer among pipe-smokers and those who smoke cigars. The chemistry of the condensates from the three main forms of tobacco smoking differs greatly and the search to find the guilty chemical goes on. But there may be a dangerous paradox here. Pipe smoke and cigar smoke is much more irritant than that from cigarettes and those who have smoked only pipes or cigars tend to avoid inhalation. The cigarette smoker who turns in his distress to the "safer" habit of pipe or cigar smoking may inhale these "stronger" smokes. In these circumstances they may yet prove to be more dangerous than cigarette smoke.

The prudent man will not put these problems to the test.

In returning to the question of pollution of the ambient air there is comfort in the fact that the problem is being solved; at least in some respects.

The Clean Air Act (1956) recognized the important fact (emphasized in the Beaver Committee's report) that, in this country pollution by coal smoke was uneconomic, filthy and harmful to health. Without waiting for further proof or for the development of economic methods to deal with other pollutants such as sulphur dioxide it sought to ban smoke. The results have been spectacular.

There has been some reduction in the ambient concentrations of sulphur dioxide despite increases in emission and this is thought to be due to the fact that in the absence of a pall of smoke over cities, the sun can shine through and break up minor temperature inversions with the consequent dispersion of all pollutants (Waller, Lawther and Martin, 1969).

There are already signs of improvement in health and the improvement in cleanliness of large cities is obvious to all. There is an urgent need to continue to apply epidemiological techniques as the scene changes so that the part played by pollution in the development of chronic disease can be assessed as experimental work continues. It is hoped that as smoke is reduced progressively while abatement of pollution by SO_2 necessarily lags behind, the respective roles of particulate pollutants and gases may be discerned.

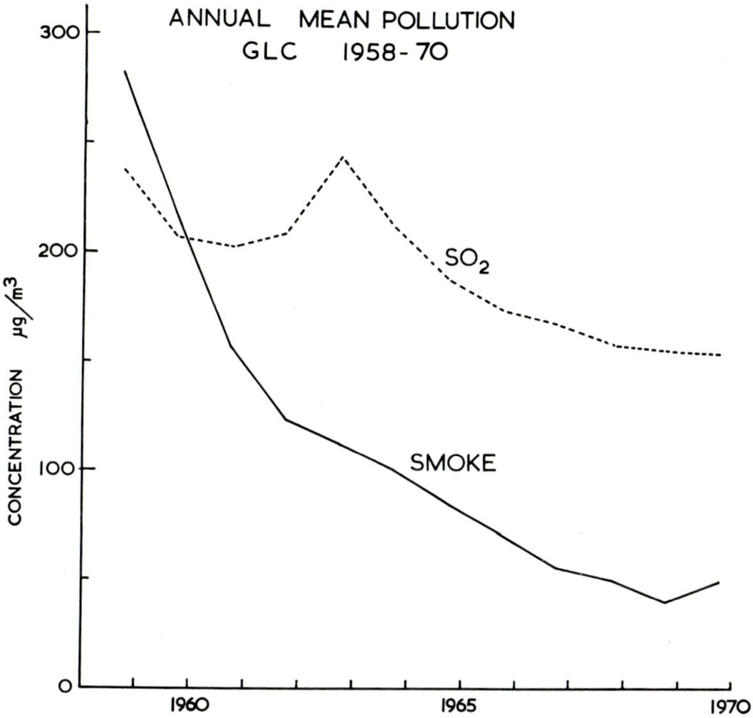

FIG. 3. Annual mean concentrations of smoke and sulphur dioxide at a group of seven sites in Inner London, 1958–70.

The old pollutants are disappearing; new pollutants, inevitably, emerge. Asbestos, once thought to be so inert and harmless can in its various forms produce serious and fatal disease; crocidolite has been shown to cause mesotheliomas of pleura and peritoneum, not only in people exposed by virtue of their occupation, but in members of the public exposed to minute doses. Beryllium is another element which was seen to cause disease in communities outside the factory. Lead and mercury are currently under attack. Not unreasonably, though often the reasons expressed are tenuous, any pollutant be it trace metal or complex organic compound, must be viewed with suspicion though not always with alarm. A proper blend of vigilance, prudence and common sense must be brought to bear on the problem of air pollution.

Industrial Bronchitis

The effects of relatively high air pollution during the working day on the health of industrial workers has been and is, the subject of much controversy. A report by a committee of the Medical Research Council (1966) concluded that the intensity of dust exposure in coal workers did not appear to be a very significant factor in the causation of chronic bronchitis. Its effects could hardly be separated from those of cigarette smoking, atmospheric pollution and socio-economic factors. Support for this general conclusion was noted in two major British investigations published since that date. Lowe (1969) has discussed the initial findings of an extensive survey in a South Wales steel works amongst men exposed to particulate airborne contaminants and to gaseous irritants such as sulphur dioxide. Although it was clear that occupation made some contribution to the initiation, progression and outcome of chronic bronchitis in the population examined, that contribution was very small compared to the effects of tobacco smoking. Rae *et al.* (1971) did find a significant relationship between the prevalence of bronchitis and the degree of exposure to airborne dust amongst miners under 44 years of age in the British Coal Industry but could not confirm this finding amongst the older men. The dominant effect of cigarette smoking was again noted in their results.

A major difficulty of surveys of this type is related to the reliability of estimates of previous exposure. Modern industrial techniques change rapidly and there are wide fluctuations in the environmental pollution produced in any one process over a period of a few years. Another difficulty lies in the measurement of the airborne dust. The use of the term "respirable dust" may prove misleading in this context. This fraction of the airborne cloud is that thought to penetrate to the alveoli and if so, is unlikely to damage the ciliated airways. The size distribution of particles causing bronchitis is unknown but is probably coarser than that defined by the respirable fraction. The respirable fraction of an airborne cloud bears no fixed relationship to the concentration of the larger particles and it is therefore inherently unlikely that a casual relationship between it and the prevalence of bronchitis could be shown. Further surveys of this aspect are now being undertaken in the mining industries of Britain and Europe.

References

Albert, R. E. and Nelson, N. (1964), "Special report to the Surgeon General's Advisory Committee on Smoking and Health."

Commins, B. T. (1969), "Formation of Polycyclic Aromatic Hydrocarbons during Pyrolysis and Combustion of Hydrocarbons." *Atmos. Environ.*, **3**, 565.

Douglas, J. W. B. and Waller, R. E. (1966), "Air Pollution and Respiratory Infection in Children." *Brit. J. Prev. Soc. Med.*, **20,** 1.

Ellison, J. McK (1965), "The Nature of Air Pollution and the Methods Available for Measuring it." *Bull Wld. Health Org.*, **32,** 399.

Ellison, J. McK. (1965), "The Particles in Town Air." *Bull. Wld. Health Org.*, **32,** 411.

Green, H. L. and Lane, W. R. (1957), "Particulate Clouds: Dusts, Smokes, and Mists; their Physics and Physical Chemistry and Industrial and Environmental Aspects." Princeton, N.J.: Van Nostrand.

Harris, W. J. (1960), "Size Distribution of Tobacco Smoke Droplets by a Replica Method." *Nature*, **186,** (4724), 537.

Horstman, S. W. and Wagman, J. "Size Analysis of Acid Aerosols by a Metal Film Technique." *Amer. Industr. Hyg. Assn. J.*, **28** (6), 523.

Lawther, P. J., Emerson, T. R. and O'Grady, F. W. (1969), "Haemophilus influenzae—Growth Stimulation by Atmosphere Pollutants." *Brit. J. Dis. Chest*, **63,** 45.

Lawther, P. J., Waller, R. E., Henderson, J. (1970), "Air Pollution and Exacerbations of Bronchitis." *Thorax*, 1970, **25** (5), 525.

Lowe, C. R. (1969), "Industrial Bronchitis." *Brit. Med. J.*, **1,** 463.

May, K. R. (1945), "The Cascade Impactor, an Instrument for Sampling Coarse Aerosols." *J. Sci. Instrum.*, **22,** 187.

Medical Research Council (1966), "Chronic Bronchitis and Occupation," *Brit. Med. J.*, **1,** 101.

Ministry of Health (1954), *Mortality and Morbidity during the London Fog of December*, 1952. No. 95—Reports on Public Health and Medical Subjects. London: H.M.S.O.

Rae, S., Walker, D. D., Attfield, M. D. (1971), "Chronic Bronchitis and Dust Exposure in British Coalminers." In *Inhaled Particles* III. Ed. W. H. Walton. London: Unwin.

Robinson, E. and Ludwig, F. L. (1967), "Particle Size Distribution of Urban Lead Aerosols." *J. Air Polln. Control Assoc.*, **17** (10), 664.

Royal College of Physicians of London (1962, 1971), "Smoking and Health, 1962; Smoking and Health Now, 1971." Pitman, London.

Waller, R. E. (1963), "Acid Droplets in Town Air." *Int. J. Air and Wat. Poll.*, **7,** 773.

Waller, R. E., Brooks, A. G. F. and Cartwright, J. (1963), "An Electron Microscope Study of Particles in Town Air." *Int. J. Air and Wat. Poll.*, **7,** 779.

Waller, R. E. and Biles, B. (1964), "The Electron Microscope in Air Pollution Research. In *Proc. 3rd Regional Conference on Electron Microscopy*. Ed. M. Tiltback. Prague: Czechoslovak Academy of Sciences, Vol. A, pp. 369–70.

Waller, R. E., Commins, B. T. and Lawther, P. J. (1964), "Air Pollution in a City Street." *Brit. J. Industr. Med.*, **22,** 128.

Waller, R. E. (1966), "The Interpretation and use of Data on Air Pollution in Epidemiological Research." *Statistician*, **16,** 45.

Waller, R. E., Lawther, P. J. and Martin, A. E. (1969), "Clean Air and Health in London." In *Proc. Clean Air Conf., Eastbourne*, 1964. Part I. London: Nat. Soc. for Clean Air, pp. 71ff.

U.S. Public Health Service (1964), *Smoking and Health.* Report of the Advisory Committee to the Surgeon General of the Public Health Service, Washington. U.S. Dept. of H. E. & W. P.H.S. Publ. No. 1, 103, 387 pp.

U.S. National Clearinghouse for Smoking and Health. *The Health Consequences of Smoking, a Public Health Service Review:* 1967. Washington U.S. Dept. of Health, Education and Welfare, Public Health Service, 1964. Supplementary Editions 1968 and 1969.

Chapter 3

Inhaled Microbes

R. E. O. Williams

Inhalation is probably the route by which pathogenic microbes most frequently enter the human body, at least in the temperate regions of the world. Such inhalation may result in immediate rejection of the microbe, or in no more than a transient and symptomless colonization of the mucosa of the upper respiratory tract; it may lead to invasion and the development of disease in upper or lower respiratory tract, or it may be followed by spread of infection to remote parts of the body. In this chapter we shall discuss the pathogenesis of the principal diseases thought to arise from inhalation, with special reference to the studies, already discussed in Chapter 1, of the way in which particles penetrate into the respiratory tract. An understanding of these aspects of "mode of spread" is essential if one is to make any rational attempt at control by methods of environmental hygiene.

It is first necessary to discuss the sources of airborne pathogenic microbes and the way in which clouds of infective particles are generated.

Sources of Infection

For almost all of the inhalation infections of man, the source of the infective particles is another man, and it seems that the route of infection is generally directly man-to-man rather than through the mediation of inanimate reservoirs.

Human sources of airborne infection. As human sources we have to recognize both those persons who have, or have had, an overt infection and those who are symptomless carriers of the pathogenic microbe.

The most obvious way in which airborne particles are generated is by sneezing, coughing and talking, during which droplets of saliva are atomized and projected into the air. This form of dispersal has received a great deal of study. During quiet breathing virtually no particles are dispersed from the nose and mouth. Sneezing produces by far the largest number, coughing fewer and talking, in most individuals, fewer still. In all these activities droplets of a wide range of particle sizes are ejected, ranging from 1 micron to 1 millimeter (Duguid, 1946; Loudon and Roberts, 1967). Whether or not an individual particle will contain a living microbe will, of course, depend on the concentration of microbes in the saliva or nasal secretion; only a small proportion of the droplets less than 5 μ in diameter can contain pathogenic microbes, but this is offset by the fact that, in the spray generated in sneezing particularly, a very large number of small droplets are liberated.

During sneezing, the salivary pool in the front of the mouth is the source of the great majority of the droplets expelled into the air, but substantial numbers of particles are also emitted from the nose and these are presumably the vehicle of spread of the common cold virus, which is only scantily present in saliva (Buckland, Bynoe and Tyrrell, 1965).

In the early years of the century Flügge, using air sampling methods now known to be very inefficient for the collection of the smaller airborne particles, showed that the range of the droplet spray around a disperser was about 2 metres. In the 1930's W. F. Wells, having devised a more efficient air sampling instrument, pointed out that the droplets in a mouth spray that are less than about 100 μ in diameter quickly evaporate to give residual nuclei of solids, including any contained bacteria; these, having a settling rate corresponding to a particle size of less than 10 μ in diameter, remain suspended in the air for long periods, and can therefore be carried some distance on turbulent air currents (see Wells, 1955). Wells' writings almost suggested that there were two quite distinct populations of particles arising from a mouth spray—droplets and droplet nuclei—but the few direct observations that have been made of the size of bacteria-carrying particles in such a spray indicate a unimodal size distribution with a mode in the region of 10–14 μ equivalent particle diameter (Lidwell, Noble and Dolphin, 1959). Size grading of the airborne particles carrying microbes in various occupied places have also yielded unimodal distributions (Table 1, and Noble, Lidwell and Kingston, 1963), and only a very small fraction of the bacteria derived from human sources are associated with particles having equivalent diameters of less than 4 μ.

Table 1

The sizes of airborne bacteria- and fungus-carrying particles
(after Noble *et al.*, 1963)

Microbe	*Place of study*	*Mean equivalent particle diameter* μ	*Interquartile range* μ
Mouth streptococci	Offices	10	4–16
Staphylococcus aureus	Hospital wards	13	8–18
Clostridium welchii	Hospital wards	11	4–18
Aspergillus fumigatus	Hospital wards	3	3–3
Candida albicans	Hospital wards	13	5–21
Trichophyton mentagrophytes	Hospital clinic	16	11–22

Note: The equivalent particle diameter is the diameter of a sphere of unit density having the same settling rate as the observed microbe-carrying particle. The original paper should be consulted for a discussion of the limitations of the estimates.

During the last few years we have recognized the importance of another route by which respiratory tract bacteria can be dispersed into the air; this is by preliminary transfer from the respiratory tract to the skin and subsequent dispersal thence on desquamated skin particles. This route has been especially well demonstrated for the staphylococci (Noble and Davies, 1965). The quantities of bacteria dispersed from the skin in quite simple activities are remarkable: Noble and Davies found some individuals to liberate over 10^6 bacteria-carrying particles while undressing and redressing in a 2-minute period. The type of clothing worn makes little difference to the numbers dispersed, and many carriers liberate large numbers while exercising naked; washing the skin with soap and water often increases the numbers liberated (Speers *et al.*, 1965).

Environmental and Animal Sources of Airborne Infection

Bacteria from human sources often contaminate secondary environmental reservoirs such as floor dust and bedclothes. Shaking bedclothes redisperses large numbers of bacteria into the air but extensive redispersal from floor dust is probably relatively unimportant unless the floors are swept with dry brooms.

Although man is by far the most important source of inhaled pathogens there are some other sources that must be mentioned. For some diseases the source is some infected animal tissues or excreta: inhalation anthrax is generally attributable to spores from infected wool and hair, and Q fever can certainly be spread through the air from infected animals by contaminated dust particles from hides, straw or placentae (Lennette and Welsh, 1951).

Pseudomonas aeruginosa (*pyocyanea*) may contaminate the water in humidifiers, both in air conditioning systems and in breathing machines and can then be inhaled and produce disease in susceptible tissues.

The fungus *Histoplasma capsulatum* flourishes in bird droppings and its spores are liberated into the air when the dried droppings are disturbed.

Lastly there are some fungi, notably *Aspergillus* spp., that are saprophytes normally present in soil; these are frequently inhaled, though they only give rise to disease in very special circumstances.

Inhalation Infections

In Table 2 there are listed the principal diseases thought to arise from inhalation infection. It will be useful to discuss the way in which some of these are thought to be spread.

Infections with invasion from the lower respiratory tract. The first group of diseases to be considered are those for which there is evidence for spread by particles small enough to penetrate into the lower respiratory

Table 2

Principal inhalation infections

Infections presumed to originate from invasion of lower respiratory tract
- Pulmonary tuberculosis
- Inhalation anthrax
- Histoplasmosis, coccidioidomycosis and aspergillosis
- ? Measles
- ? Chickenpox

Infections presumed to originate from invasion of upper respiratory tract
- Common cold
- Streptococcal sore throat
- Diphtheria

Infections with doubtful portal of entry
- Pneumonia
- Whooping cough
- Meningococcal meningitis
- Respiratory virus infections

tract. For one of these diseases—pulmonary tuberculosis—such deep penetration is probably essential; for the others there is certainly the possibility of upper respiratory tract infection as well.

Tuberculosis. Several experimental studies in animals suggest that pulmonary tuberculosis arises from the inhalation of very small particles into the alveoli in depths of the lung. It is only particles of the order of 2 μ diameter or less that have a high probability of penetrating to the alveoli and it has even been suggested that it is only the smaller tubercle bacilli that are able to reach the alveoli and infect. In children, the primary infection (the "Ghon focus") is found in the area of the lung receiving the greatest ventilation; there may be subsequent secondary establishment of tubercle bacilli in the apical areas and in the lower lobes, perhaps favoured by the high oxygen tension in these areas (Stead, 1967). Some evidence that primary tuberculous lesions acquired during adult life may also be more common in the less well ventilated upper parts of the lung has been reported (R.C.P. Prophit Tuberculosis Survey, 1948).

An ingenious series of air-sampling studies in a tuberculosis hospital (Riley *et al.*, 1962) have shown quite clearly that infected patients do in fact liberate tubercle bacilli in particles that can remain airborne for a considerable period though exact sizing has not been reported. There is also some epidemiological evidence for spread of infection at a distance, although it is well known that ordinarily infection seems to require rather close contact. The explanation may be that most patients liberate relatively small numbers of infected particles of the right size. An interesting feature that emerged from Riley's studies was the great variation in the numbers of airborne particles liberated by different patients, even among those with tubercle bacilli demonstrable in their sputum.

Inhalation anthrax. "Wool-sorters' disease" results from inhalation of the spores of *Bacillus anthracis* into the lungs and their transport in lymphatics to the mediastinum, where they produce the characteristic and very serious disease. In animal experiments clouds of single spores, which can penetrate to the alveoli, are much more infective than clouds of 12 μ particles, which are retained in the upper air passages (Druett *et al.*, 1953), and it seems reasonable to suppose that the disease in man results from inhalation of particles small enough to reach at least as far as the bronchi or bronchioles. Brachman, Kaufmann and Dalldorf (1966) demonstrated large numbers of *B. anthracis* in particles estimated to have a diameter less than 5 μ in the air of a factory processing infected goat hair.

Histoplasmosis and coccidioidomycosis. These two diseases result from the inhalation of spores from fungi that are growing in soil or, in the case of histoplasmosis, bird faeces. Judging from the site of the primary lesions, they probably result from the inhalation of small particles such as spores or fragments of mycelium. Neither of these two diseases occurs in Britain; histoplasmosis is rather common throughout the United States, while coccidioidomycosis is confined to the arid areas in the southern United States.

Pulmonary aspergillosis. Spores of *Aspergillus fumigatus* are very commonly present in the air, even in cities, but this fungus only acts as a pathogen when there is some pre-existing disease of the lung, such as chronic tuberculosis with cavitation, or asthma.

Measles and chickenpox. These, with tuberculosis, represent the diseases for which there is reasonable epidemiological evidence for spread on the small airborne particles of Wells' "droplet nucleus" type. Thus there is a long and well-documented tradition of great difficulty in containing the spread of both measles and chickenpox by simple segregation in separate rooms in infectious-disease hospitals (see Williams, 1956). And, in schools, ultra-violet air disinfection seems to have some effect on the rate of spread of infection (though not to the extent of making this a useful hygienic method) (Report, 1954; Wells, 1955). Both diseases are especially infective in the early catarrhal stage and presumably the virus is present in saliva in concentrations sufficient to yield infective droplets that desiccate to particles of 10 μ diameter or less. Chickenpox, in contrast to smallpox, does not seem to be spread by infected skin squames or scabs.

There is no direct evidence on the preferred site of invasion in the respiratory tract.

Infections with Invasion from the Upper Respiratory Tract

Common cold. The principal reservoir of virus in the infected person is certainly the nose and throat. Experimental studies with volunteers infected with a coxsackievirus A21, which produces colds, have shown that infection can be conveyed by airborne droplets, and that the infection is established better from nasal deposition than from small droplets inhaled into the lungs (see Tyrrell, 1967). Moreover virus probably survives better in large droplets than in small. All these studies are consonant with epidemiological observations, which suggest that the spread of the disease occurs most readily among persons who are in relatively close contact (Tyrrell, 1965), and is probably rarely due to the long-distance spread that might be mediated by droplet nuclei. There is no good evidence that the virus survives desiccation well enough to permit spread by fomites.

There is now good epidemiological evidence that the incidence of colds is directly related to periods of cold weather (Lidwell, Morgan and Williams, 1965) but the reason for this is not known.

It has also been shown for the common cold, as for streptococcal infections and pulmonary tuberculosis, that some carriers are able to disseminate enormously more virus than others.

Streptococcal sore throat and diphtheria. These are two diseases for which it is reasonable to postulate airborne spread on particles of a size trapped in the nose or throat; deposition on the nasal mucous membrane can certainly be followed by transport on the mucous blanket to the tonsillar region. Diphtheria had largely disappeared as an important epidemic disease by the time that any precise studies of mode of spread had become possible, but it is very probable that it would behave in a very similar way to the streptococcal infections.

We have the impression, from various studies, that infection takes place largely at relatively short range, and studies in the U.S. Armed Forces indicated a substantial reduction in infection rate with increasing distance separating the beds of infected and susceptible men in a dormitory (Wannamaker, 1954).

There is very good evidence that persons who harbour streptococci in the nose disperse far more of the bacteria into the environment than those who carry them only in the throat (Hamburger *et al.*, 1945); it may be that this is associated with a greater liability to skin carriage, though this has not been established.

Streptococci (and diphtheria bacilli) survive very well in floor dust and on fabrics and can often be found in very large numbers in the environment of infected patients and of some healthy carriers. This has naturally led to the idea that dust can act as an important reservoir of infection. On the other hand there is some evidence that the streptococci in dust lack virulence (Rammelkamp *et al.*, 1958). Attempts to demonstrate the importance of this route of infection by methods designed to control floor- and fabric-dust have given very variable results but the general feeling is now that, although streptococci from the environment can on occasion give rise to infection, this is probably far less common than their frequency in the environment might suggest.

Staphylococcal nasal carriage. Although *Staphylococcus aureus* rarely produces disease in the nose or throat, symptomless carriage in the anterior nares is very common and is especially important in hospital as the way in which the endemic, antibiotic-resistant strains are maintained. Nasal carriers act as a succession of reservoirs from which wound and other infections can arise.

Nasal carriers of staphylococci very commonly contaminate their skin and in some people there is certainly multiplication of the staphylococci on or in the skin. It is the carriers who harbour the greatest numbers of staphylococci on the skin who disperse them most readily into the environment (Solberg, 1965) and it seems that the airborne staphylococci are usually attached to skin squames; these are flakes of skin commonly about 30 μ across, but because of their flat shape they behave in air as if they were spheres with a diameter about 14 μ.

The fact that staphylococci, like haemolytic streptococci, survive well in the environment has encouraged the idea that floor and blanket dust, which often yield staphylococci in large numbers, must be important reservoirs for infection. However, virtually all controlled attempts have failed to demonstrate any benefit from measures designed to reduce infection from blankets. This may be explained in two ways. On the one hand clean blankets put on the bed of a disperser become heavily contaminated within a very short time and, on the other hand, friction between the skin and any fabric distributes skin bacteria into the air; it may well be that the contribution of the blanket itself to the aerial load is often relatively unimportant.

The importance of the aerial route of spread is demonstrable by the fact that the rate of acquisition of carriage in hospital can be influenced by air movement; when there is little air exchange between the areas in which patients are nursed, the nasal cross-infection rate is low (Lidwell *et al.*, 1966). Nasal colonization by staphylococci is one of the very few situations where we might be able to make some estimate of the average infecting dose. Lidwell and his colleagues estimated, from studies in a surgical ward, that an inhaled dose of 10 airborne staphylococcal particles corresponded to a probable risk of nasal acquisition of 1:300 to 1:800.

Infections with Doubtful Portal of Invasion

Pneumonia. Pneumococcal pneumonia is an acute exogenous infection in which the disease starts in the alveoli; it might be thought therefore to be a disease arising from the inhalation of bacteria attached to very small particles. Animal experiments have indeed shown that pneumonia can be initiated by the introduction of *Streptococcus pneumoniae* in droplets of mucus into the alveoli. However, it seems more likely that the natural disease arises by preliminary colonization of the nasopharynx with the pneumococci, followed by their transfer—perhaps by inhalation—to the lungs (see Nungester and Klepser, 1938). There are no really useful studies of the way in which this infection spreads from person to person.

Whooping cough. In whooping cough due to *Bordetella pertussis* the principal sites of infection are the small bronchi and bronchioles but there is certainly also colonization of the nasopharynx; whether the nasopharyngeal colonization represents the primary site of infection, or whether it is secondary to the airway infection is not known.

Meningococcal meningitis is another example of a disease in which there is nasopharyngeal colonization though the centre of the disease is elsewhere in the body. It seems clear that, in this case, the nasopharynx is the primary site of infection, and that transfer to the meninges is usually by the blood stream, although spread along the arachnoid sheaths surrounding the olfactory nerves as they penetrate the ethmoid bone cannot be ruled out.

Epidemics of meningococcal meningitis have notoriously occurred in circumstances of severe overcrowding, as in military barracks. Probably the infection is conveyed by droplets from the mouth and throat, which are deposited on or conveyed to the nasopharynx. Artenstein and Lamson (1970) have shown that some carriers can disperse more than 100 meningococci in a single cough. They emphasize the fact that healthy carriers commonly far outnumber patients with overt disease and that, in a military population, sleeping quarters form an important but by no means the only area in which transmission takes place.

Respiratory virus infections. There can be no doubt that influenza and other virus infections of the respiratory tract are spread by the airborne route. Experiments with adenoviruses have shown that lung infections can often be produced more readily with small-droplet aerosols than with large (Couch *et al.*, 1966), so it may be assumed that the febrile lower respiratory tract infections may be conveyed on small particles that are deposited in the depths of the lung.

Other virus infections. Smallpox is widely thought to be spread by inhalation and the virus can certainly survive in the crusts and on contaminated fabrics. There is a suggestion that, as dispersed from the upper respiratory tract the virus tends to be associated with the larger airborne particles, which would imply deposition on the upper respiratory tract. There are, however, a number of reasonably well attested anecdotes indicating that, on occasion, the virus can be spread through a considerable distance, which could be achieved only by small airborne particles.

Poliomyelitis and infective hepatitis are two virus infections that are generally spread by the faecal-oral route but probably can sometimes be contracted by inhalation.

Control of Inhalation Infection

From what has been said already it will be clear that the current belief is that, with certain exceptions, most inhalation infections can arise from the particles large enough to be trapped in the upper respiratory tract and that such epidemiological evidence as is available suggests that short-range infection is more common than long-range. This is important when we come to consider the methods available for controlling the spread of infection.

The importance of long-range airborne spread of infection has been very variously assessed over the years and this has been reflected in the use of widely varying methods for the control of the spread of disease. At one extreme was Grancher's plan for isolating children simply by enclosing them in a wire-netting cage to prevent transfer by fomites; at the other extreme is the construction of isolation hospitals consisting of single-bedroom wards all opening on to a verandah. Various methods of chemical and physical air disinfection have also been advocated.

The control methods that need to be discussed include: air disinfection, dilution-ventilation, directional ventilation, and the control of the sources of airborne microbes.

Air disinfection. Four air disinfectants have been submitted to reasonably adequate testing: ultra-violet irradiation, triethylene glycol, hexyl resorcinol and α-hydroxy-α-methyl-butyric acid ("C acid").

Ultra-violet cannot be used for direct irradiation of the air of an occupied room because of the ease with which conjunctivitis results from looking at the lamps. Wells devised the method of irradiating the air in the upper part of a room and relying on natural air turbulence to carry the airborne microbes into the irradiated zone. Upper-air irradiation has been extensively tested for the control of infection in school rooms (Wells, Wells and Wilder, 1942; Report, 1954). In the latter trials the irradiation reduced the air count of mouth bacteria, used as an "indicator" for respiratory tract pathogens, by about 75% but had much less effect on the general bacterial flora which are mostly derived from skin and clothing dust. In both American and British experience there was a reduction in the rate of spread of measles and, in the former at least, of chickenpox, though the ultimate attack rate was not usefully affected. There was no clear effect on any other infection. There does not appear to be any case for the use of ultra-violet as an air disinfectant for occupied rooms.

Ultra-violet has also been employed as a disinfectant "curtain" in the doorways to isolation rooms and some workers have reported that this has reduced the spread of infection, though none of the trials has been really adequately controlled. The principle of direct irradiation has also been used in surgical operating rooms, all occupants of the rooms being provided with protective clothing and eye shades. A large-scale controlled trial revealed very little advantage for the method (Nat. Res. Counc., 1964).

Extensive tests were made of triethylene glycol as an air disinfectant in the United States during World War II, but although some encouraging results were obtained, the overall conclusion must be that this is not a useful method for controlling airborne infection (Williams, 1960).

Fewer trials have been made of hexyl resorcinol or C acid but our own investigations of both these substances were very discouraging (Kingston, Lidwell and Williams, 1962).

One major difficulty in the use of all methods of air disinfection appears to be the impossibility of attaining a sufficiently high rate of kill of airborne bacteria. But it also seems to be the case that the air disinfectants are more active on the small airborne particles than the large. Perhaps this, and the fact that so many of the infections are spread at such short range that air disinfectants have no opportunity to act, accounts for the lack of clinical effect.

Dilution ventilation. An obvious alternative to killing microbes within a room is to remove them by dilution with fresh air, that is by an increase in the air-change rate. There is a venerable tradition—in Britain at least—that an increase in the supply of fresh air is "healthy" and it has often been postulated that the seasonal variations in respiratory tract infections are attributable to the alterations in air change rates imposed by the variations in external temperature. Facts are unfortunately very hard to come by. Air-change rates undoubtedly do vary with season, as does the incidence of the common cold, but one attempt to decrease the incidence of colds by increase in ventilation had no demonstrable effect (Kingston, Lidwell and Williams, 1962). The trouble may well be, as with chemical air disinfection, that practicable increases in ventilation rate are insufficient to reduce the concentration of airborne microbes by the amount needed to yield a demonstrable reduction in attack rate, for the slope of the dose-response line may be small (as it is with the acquisition of staphylococci in the nose, see Lidwell *et al.*, 1966, 1970). At the same time, if it is a fact that most infections result from the inhalation of the larger airborne particles, conveyed at relatively short range, then one would not expect a great result from increase in ventilation.

Directional ventilation. When the problem is to control the spread of airborne microbes from one room to another rather than from one person to another within the same room, it is sometimes possible to use differential air pressures. This has been extensively discussed in relation to the protection of surgical operating rooms, and there is now a considerable body of experience indicating that "positive pressure" ventilation of such areas reduces the incidence of post-operative wound infection (see Williams *et al.*, 1966).

The same principle has been used in the design of isolation wards and there is some evidence that the rate of acquisition of nasal carriage of *Staph. aureus* can be reduced by this means (Williams *et al.*, 1959). However, recent studies by Lidwell and his colleagues (1966) suggest that a very large reduction in the numbers of organisms inhaled will be needed to effect any large reduction in the acquisition rate. It has also been found that it is difficult to obtain really satisfactory isolation of adjacent spaces by air pressure differences. All this indicates the need for more observations on this topic.

A recent development in methods of "directional ventilation" is the use of high volumes of ventilating air introduced into the room in such a way as to give a uni-directional or "laminar" air flow. The direction of the air flow can be vertical or horizontal, but the horizontal method is the one generally preferred for hospital use and has been tested in surgical operating rooms (Whitcomb and Clapper, 1966 and see Scott, 1970) and in an intensive therapy ward (Lidwell and Towers, 1969). There is no doubt that laminar flow ventilation systems have given substantial control of airborne transfer of bacteria within the ventilated space and they may well have a useful place when it is such transfer that has to be guarded against. The proper place of these systems, however, can only be established by much more work.

Control of sources. The exclusion of the source of infection from contact with susceptibles may seem the ideal method of control. In fact it is often difficult to operate usefully. With measles, chickenpox and tuberculosis, the patients are infective before they develop signs of disease and indeed with measles have often almost reached the end of the infective period before the disease is diagnosed. Although this is not the case with tuberculosis, the patients may have been infective for so long before detection that most of the susceptibles among their immediate contacts are already infected (see Fox, 1968).

Moreover the really active dispersers of infection may be recognized only by bacteriological examination, as for example with staphylococcal or streptococcal carriers. With the staphylococcus there is the additional complication that it is not really possible to distinguish the few carriers of dangerous strains from the very numerous carriers of relatively harmless strains. Similarly with the meningococcus or pneumococcus the great majority of infections are symptomless, so that exclusion of sources is impracticable.

Great efforts have been expended on controlling the dispersal of bacteria especially streptococci and staphylococci from floor dust and from factories, but conclusive evidence that this reduces the incidence of infection has not been obtained.

On the other hand, it ought to be possible to prevent all pseudomonas infections arising from contaminated breathing machines by eliminating the bacteria from the machine, though the design of many current machines makes this aim difficult to achieve. One of the factors responsible for the decrease in inhalation anthrax in this century has probably been the disinfection of imported wool. But there is little hope of preventing histoplasmosis or coccidioidomycosis by controlling the source.

Water was virtually eliminated as a major route for the transfer of infection 50 years ago and in the subsequent years there has been great progress in the control of food-borne infection. In contrast there are few areas in which air hygiene can claim to have reduced the incidence of disease; the decline of many of the inhalation diseases discussed in this chapter has been due to other factors, including, of course, the reduction in overcrowding of dwellings. The reasons for the relative ineffectiveness of air hygiene are now clear: first that so many of the infections are conveyed at short range, and, second, that air is difficult to manipulate or to sterilize in ordinary conditions of living or working.

References

Artenstein, M. S. and Lamson, T. (1970), "Meningococcal Transmission among Army Recruits. " In Aerobiology, p. 1. Ed. I. H. Silver. London: Academic Press.

Brachman, P. S., Kaufmann, A. F. and Dalldorf, F. G. (1966), "Industrial Inhalation Anthrax." *Bact. Rev.*, **30,** 646.

Buckland, F. E., Bynoe, M. L. and Tyrrell, D. A. J. (1965), "Experiments on the Spread of Colds. II. Studies in Volunteers with Coxsackievirus A21." *J. Hyg., Camb.*, **63,** 327.

Couch, R. B., Cate, T. R., Fleet, W. F., Gerone, P. J. and Knight, V. (1966), "Aerosol-induced Adenoviral Illness Resembling the Naturally Occurring Illness in Military Recruits." *Am. Rev. resp. Dis.*, **93,** 529.

Druett, H. A., Henderson, D. W., Packman, L. and Peacock, S. (1953), "Studies on Respiratory Infection. I. The Influence of Particle Size on Respiratory Infection with Anthrax Spores." *J. Hyg., Camb.*, **51,** 359.

Duguid, J. P. (1946), "The Size and the Duration of Air-carriage of Respiratory Droplets and Droplet-nuclei." *J. Hyg., Camb.*, **44,** 471.

Fox, W. (1968), "The Chemotherapy of Tuberculosis in Developing Countries." In *Recent Advances in Respiratory Tuberculosis*, p. 127. 6th edn. Ed. F. Heaf and N. Lloyd Rusby. London: J. & A. Churchill.

Hamburger, M., Jr., Green, Margaret, J. and Hamburger, Virginia G. (1945), "The Problem of the 'Dangerous Carrier' of Hemolytic Streptococci. II. Spread of Infection by Individuals with Strongly Positive Nose Cultures who Expelled Large Numbers of Hemolytic Streptococci." *J. infect. Dis.*, **77,** 96.

Kingston, D., Lidwell, O. M. and Williams, R. E. O. (1962), "The Epidemiology of the Common Cold. III. The Effect of Ventilation, Air Disinfection and Room Size." *J. Hyg., Camb.*, **60,** 341.

Lennette, E. H. and Welsh, H. H. (1951), "Q Fever in California. X. Recovery of *Coxiella Burneti* from the Air of Premises Harboring Infected Goats." *Am. J. Hyg.*, **54,** 44.

Lidwell, O. M., Morgan, R. W. and Williams, R. E. O. (1965), "The Epidemiology of the Common Cold. IV. The Effect of Weather." *J. Hyg., Camb.*, **63,** 427.

Lidwell, O. M., Noble, W. C. and Dolphin, G. W. (1959), "The Use of Radiation to Estimate the Numbers of Micro-organisms in Air-borne Particles." *J. Hyg., Camb.*, **57,** 299.

Lidwell, O. M., Polakoff, Sheila, Jevons, M. Patricia, Parker, M. T., Shooter, R. A., French, Valentine I. and Dunkerley, D. R. (1966), "Staphylococcal Infection in Thoracic Surgery: Experience in a Subdivided Ward." *J. Hyg., Camb.*, **64,** 321.

Lidwell, O. M., Polakoff, Sheila, Davies, J., Hewitt, J. H., Shooter, R. A., Walker, K. A., Gaya, H. and Taylor, G. W. (1970), "Nasal Acquisition of Staphylococcus aureus in a Subdivided and Mechanically Ventilated Ward: Endemic Prevalence of a Single Staphylococcal Strain." *J. Hyg., Camb.*, **68,** 417.

Lidwell, O. M. and Towers, A. G. (1969), "Protection from Microbial Contamination in a Room Ventilated by a Uni-directional Air Flow." *J. Hyg. Camb.*, **67,** 95.

Loudon, R. G. and Roberts, Rena M. (1967), "Droplet Expulsion from the Respiratory Tract." *Am. Rev. resp. Dis.*, **95,** 435.

National Research Council (1964), "Postoperative Wound Infections: the Influence of Ultraviolet Irradiation of the Operating Room and of Various Other Factors." *Ann. Surg.*, **160,** suppl.

Noble, W. C. and Davies, R. R. (1965), "Studies on the Dispersal of Staphylococci." *J. clin. Path.*, **18,** 16.

Noble, W. C., Lidwell, O. M. and Kingston, D. (1963), "The Size Distribution of Airborne Particles Carrying Micro-organisms." *J. Hyg., Camb.*, **61,** 385.

Nungester, W. J. and Klepser, R. G. (1938), "A Possible Mechanism of Lowered Resistance to Pneumonia." *J. infect. Dis.*, **63,** 94.

Rammelkamp, C. H., Jr., Morris, A. J., Catanzaro, F. J., Wannamaker, L. W., Chamovitz, R. and Marple, E. C. (1958), "Transmission of Group A Streptococci. III. The Effect of Drying on the Infectivity of the Organism for Man." *J. Hyg., Camb.*, **56,** 280.

Report (1954), Air Hygiene Committee, Medical Research Council, *Air Disinfection with Ultra-violet Irradiation. Its Effect on Illness Among School-children.* M.R.C. Spec. Rep. Ser. No. 283.

Riley, R. L., Mills, C. C., O'Grady, F., Sultan, L. U., Wittstadt, F. and Shivpuri, D. N. (1962), "Infectiousness of Air from a Tuberculosis Ward. Ultraviolet Irradiation of Infected Air: Comparative Infectiousness of Different Patients." *Am. Rev. resp. Dis.*, **85,** 511.

Royal College of Physicians (1948), *Tuberculosis in Young Adults—Report on Prophit Tuberculosis Survey*, 1935–1944. By M. Daniels, F. Ridehalgh and V. H. Springett. London: H. K. Lewis.

Scott, C. C. (1970), "Laminar/linear Flow System of Ventilation." *Lancet*, **1,** 989–992.

Solberg, C. O. (1965), "A Study of Carriers of *Staphylococcus aureus*." *Acta med. scand.*, **178,** Suppl. 436.

Speers, R., Jr., Bernard, H., O'Grady, F. and Shooter, R. A. (1965), "Increased Dispersal of Skin Bacteria into the Air after Shower-baths." *Lancet*, **1,** 478.

Stead, W. W. (1967), "Pathogenesis of a First Episode of Chronic Pulmonary Tuberculosis in Man: Recrudescence of Residuals of the Primary Infection or Exogenous Reinfection?" *Am. Rev. resp. Dis.*, **95,** 729.

Tyrrell, D. A. J. (1965), *Common Colds and Related Diseases.* London: Edward Arnold.

Tyrrell, D. A. J. (1967), "The Spread of Viruses of the Respiratory Tract by the Airborne Route." In *Airborne Microbes*, p. 286. Ed. by P. H. Gregory and J. L. Monteith. Cambridge University Press.

Wannamaker, L. W. (1954), "The Epidemiology of Streptococcal Infections." In *Streptococcal Infections*, p. 157. Ed. M. McCarty. New York: Columbia University Press.

Wells, W. F. (1955), *Airborne Contagion and Air Hygiene. An Ecological Study of Droplet Infections*. Cambridge, Mass.: Harvard University Press.

Wells, W. F., Wells, M. W. and Wilder, T. S. (1942), "The Environmental Control of Epidemic Contagion. I. An Epidemiologic Study of Radiant Disinfection of Air in Day Schools." *Am. J. Hyg.*, **35,** 97.

Whitcomb, J. G. and Clapper, W. E. (1966), "Ultraclean Operating Room." *Am. J. Surg.*, **112,** 681.

Williams, R. E. O. (1956), "The Progress of Ideas on Hospital Infection." *Bull. Hyg.*, **31,** 965.

Williams, R. E. O. (1960), "Intramural Spread of Bacteria and Viruses in Human Populations." *Ann. Rev. Microbiol.*, **14,** 43.

Williams, R. E. O., Blowers, R., Garrod, L. P. and Shooter, R. A. (1966), *Hospital Infection: Causes and Prevention.* 2nd edn. London: Lloyd-Luke (Medical Books) Ltd.

Williams, R. E. O., Jevons, M. Patricia, Shooter, R. A., Hunter, C. J. W., Girling, J. A., Griffiths, J. D. and Taylor, G. W. (1959), "Nasal Staphylococci and Sepsis in Hospital Patients." *Br. med. J.*, **2,** 658.

Chapter 4

Airborne Allergens

D. C. F. Muir

The respiratory tract is the main route whereby extrinsic antigens of clinical importance gain access to the body. The atmosphere is now known to contain a host of airborne particles in concentrations, which, although harmless to most human subjects and animals, are associated with clinical symptoms in some individuals. A subject's response depends mainly on his immunological reactivity but also on the nature and quantity of the inhaled material and on the size, shape and density of the particles. So complex is the variety of these floating particles in the air that the identification of specific causal relationships between any one fraction and the severity of symptoms in an individual present formidable problems. This is particularly so in bronchial asthma where multiple sensitivity is often present and the allergic component but one aetiological factor in a disease which may change in character over a period of years. The minute quantity of antigens which is able to provoke symptoms in some circumstances, and the absence of any experimental technique for their investigation other than by the laborious one of clinical trial underline the remarkable progress that has been made in this direction. The fact that most of the population remains healthy, and that even atopic asthmatics do not wheeze all the time is, in itself, remarkable since it is quite certain that both groups continuously inhale huge numbers of potentially antigenic particles throughout their lives.

The Environment in the Home

The most difficult of all airborne clouds to characterize and, at the same time, that which is probably the most important cause of allergic symptoms is to be found in the air of a patient's home. This is the dust encountered by the new-born infant taking its first breath and the one to which it will be exposed during each succeeding day. The dust contains fractions of every material associated with life in the home. It arises from carpets, curtains, clothing, bedding, dander or skin debris of human origin, hair and dander from dogs, cats and other household pets, horsehair or feathers from pillows and mattresses, food debris and many more sources. Most of this material cannot be identified or measured in samples of dust collected in a room, and exposure must be inferred from the proximity of possible sources within the house. Since Floyer in 1698 described the provocation of allergic symptoms by house dust it has been recognized that such dust is of particular importance in allergy, and strenuous efforts have been made to isolate the specific components responsible for symptoms. Samples of dust have been collected and examined on many occasions, and some general conclusions may be drawn. Pollen grains, for example, unless plants are actually in the home, can only enter from outside the house. Indoor pollen-counts therefore tend to reflect the general pattern of the outdoor spora, but in very much lower concentrations. In dry houses the fungal spores of the air, chiefly *Cladosporium herbarium* in summer and *Penicillium Spp.* in winter, are also derived mainly from external sources although again present in considerably lower concentrations (Richards, 1954; Adams and Hyde, 1965). After shaking bedding or clothing, however, huge concentrations of spores become airborne (Maunsell, 1952). In damp houses there may be heavy fungal growths on floors or wallpaper, and the airborne spores reflect the dominant species in each room. The possibility that insects might constitute the main allergic component of house-dust was suggested by Dekker (1928) and again by Voorhorst *et al.* (1964) who found large numbers of the acarine mite *Dermatophagoides*, particularly the species *D. pteronyssinus*, in the dust of mattresses. The mite is about 300 μ long and feeds on keratin derived from flock, hair, feathers and above all from human skin or dander. The last presumably accounts for its particular presence in the dust of pillows, bed linen and mattresses. These different sources of keratin serve as food for the mite, and its presence in each may account for their common antigenic properties on clinical testing (Frankland *et al.*, 1970). The mite grows best in conditions of high relative humidity at a temperature of about 25° C and is most abundant between the months of September and November. Although found in greater numbers in dust from damp houses by Spieksma (1967), this was not confirmed by Maunsell *et al.* (1968) in dust collected from mattresses in various types of house, and they suggested that the microclimate of the mattresses examined was as important as that of the house itself. The mite may become airborne, and concentrations of about 1 mite in 5 cubic metres of air were noted during bed-making by Cunnington and Gregory (1968). The airborne concentrations of insect debris and faecal pellets which are also allergenic are unknown. The sensitivity of the mite to humidity makes it unable to breed in homes in mountainous areas where mite asthma does not occur. The external air is very cold in these regions and, as a result, contains negligible water vapour. On being heated within the home the relative humidity of the air falls to an exceedingly low level although the use of artificial humidifiers may alter this situation.

The Outdoor Environment

Kirkman first observed in 1835 that grass pollen could cause hay fever. Since that date an extensive literature has appeared on the particulate content of the outdoor atmosphere. The possibility of identifying individual pollen grains and fungal spores by microscopy makes them more amenable to study than the amorphous dust from the interior of houses. The general pollution of cities is, of course, equally difficult to categorize but is fortunately non-allergenic. The aerobiology of the atmosphere is exceedingly complex and contains many species that may cause symptoms in sensitive subjects. It includes fungal spores, pollen grains, algae, insect and plant debris, each with its season and response to wind, temperature and rainfall. The estimation of the particulate content of the air is technically difficult. The simplest method is to expose a horizontal microscope slide for a measured interval of time and to count the pollen grains or other particles which fall on to it. Exposed culture plates may be used in the same way for counting and identifying fungal spores. Both methods have been widely used because of simplicity of the technique. Unfortunately, it may give a wholly false estimate of the relative numbers of different species. Each particle is collected in proportion to its terminal velocity (see Chapter 1) and larger particles are therefore collected preferentially. A number of correction factors have been derived to adjust the results but these are unsatisfactory. This is because the collection efficiency of an exposed horizontal surface is highly sensitive to the direction and velocity of the wind which may vary from one moment to another.

The gravity-slide technique does give an accurate estimate of the seasons at which individual pollens are released into the atmosphere, however. In another sense the biased collection of large particles is less misleading than it appears. Hyde and Adams (1960) pointed out that the actual dose of an allergen reaching the respiratory tract depends on the total mass of material in the air and not solely on the numerical concentration of the particles, without regard to their individual size. Nevertheless, very small particles are likely to be missed altogether by the gravity-slide, and it is only since the introduction of more accurate methods that the high concentrations of *Urtica* (Nettle) and of *Sporobolomyces* (Shadow yeast) in the air have been appreciated. Several instruments for this purpose have been described, and the Hirst (1952) spore trap is widely used. Measured volumes of air are drawn through a narrow slit situated in front of a sticky microscope slide or band. The particulate matter in the air is impacted on the slide which is examined later. The trap has a high collection efficiency but this falls to about 50% in the case of particles of 3 μ in diameter. Nevertheless, an error of this size is very small compared to that of previous methods. Particles of about 1 μ in diameter are not collected accurately, and there may also be errors due to the technical difficulty of ensuring that a representative sample of the larger particles enter the slit. Instruments for the accurate determination of the concentrations of large particles and which are also independent of wind speed are described by Harrington (1959).

Thommen (1931) summarized early knowledge on the pollen content of the air and observed that high concentrations of these particles were characteristic of the wind-pollinated or anemophilous plants. Such plants constitute about 10% of all species and contain all the important plant allergens. The individual grains are produced in vast quantities and are small enough to remain airborne for a considerable time. They are smooth and spherical, and form a dry powder, easily dispersed by the wind which may carry them far from the point of origin. The flowers are inconspicuous and contrast sharply with the showy blossoms popular in garden flowers which, being insect-pollinated, contribute little airborne pollen to the environment and are therefore relatively unimportant in allergy. The anemophilous plants may be either trees, grasses or herbaceous weeds. Each group has a characteristic pollination season.

Many surveys of airborne allergens have been made in Britain using the older gravity slide and the Hirst trap. A complete outline of these has been published by Hyde (1969). The grass pollens in these investigations are grouped together for convenience since they have antigenic similarities, but each species of tree, plant and fungus is considered separately.

Tree pollen is shed in early spring before the foliage is developed. The season is fairly short and lasts only seven to twenty-one days. In southern Britain it lasts from May to early June. The most widespread trees are the oak, ash, elm, beech, birch and alder. Cities may have special tree populations such as the plane trees of London. Plane trees rarely cause allergic symptoms, however, and trees generally are uncommon causes of pollenosis. Hyde (1956) demonstrated wide fluctuations in the yearly concentrations of individual species. These fluctuations may be important in influencing the frequency with which individuals develop allergic symptoms and also make it very difficult to assess the results of desensitization therapy.

Grass pollen is the characteristic allergen of summer. High concentrations are recorded from the end of May to mid-July in England and about two weeks later in Scotland (Hyde, 1952). Although these dates refer to the main season, smaller amounts of pollen are present throughout the summer. This prolonged high exposure establishes grass pollen as the outstanding cause of hay fever in Britain. The concentration varies from season to season but not nearly so much as does that of tree-pollens.

The wind-pollinated flowers are those usually classified as "weeds". Hyde (1959) found that three types are dominant, *Plantago* (Plantain), *Urtica* (Nettle) and *Rumex* (Sorrell), but none are common causes of clinical allergy. Their seasons are longer than those of grasses or trees and extend from the end of July to the beginning of October. *Urtica* is outstanding in the length of its season (about 110 days) and in the concentration of its airborne pollen which may equal that of grass. Ragweed, the major cause of hay fever in America, is included in this group but grows in Britain only locally.

Fungal spores are generally much smaller than pollen grains but their numerical concentrations in the air may be exceedingly high. Complex methods have been evolved to facilitate their dispersal into the air, and the environmental factors controlling these release mechanisms largely determine their airborne concentrations at any given time. Being small they are widely distributed by air currents and are found in all parts of the world.

Of the fungal spores which have been identified two are now known to dominate the outdoor air of Britain—*Cladosporium herbarium* and *Sporobolomyces*. However, the majority of spores trapped from the air cannot be identified with certainty and are only classified as belonging to one of the major groups of *Ascomycetes* or *Basidiomycetes*. Most live on growing or decaying vegetation and thus reach high concentrations during the summer or autumn months. *Ascomycetes* constitute the largest group of fungi, and their spores are usually released by "explosive" discharge during moist weather. *Basidiomycetes* include toadstools and bracket fungi and are particularly common near woodlands. The winter months are relatively free of allergens with the exception of the *Aspergilli* and *Penicillia*. These reach their highest levels between October and April.

The relative concentrations of each species depend on the local vegetation, but the extensive surveys made at Cardiff have been summarized by Hyde and Adams (1960), and their main findings are shown in Figs. 1 and 2. The results are probably fairly typical of the outdoor air in Britain.

Insects are known to be highly allergenic to man. Hamilton (1959) measured the amount of insect debris in the air and found a high concentration during August and September with the maximum daily count occurring between late afternoon and dusk.

The surveys mentioned give a general indication of the content of the air over wide sections of the country, but there are special difficulties in applying the results to individual patients. A given region may be dominated by the ecology of the locality such as large woods, parks, farmlands and the proximity of rivers, estuaries and the sea. Urban developments represent a particularly important example since they contain a high proportion of the population. Blackley pointed out many years ago that the centres of large cities were relatively free of airborne pollen. Surveys of city atmospheres have usually been conducted with instruments on the roofs of buildings, but Davies (1965) has shown that such instruments probably sample air blown in from the surrounding countryside. The air at street level may be totally different and is likely to be dominated by local sources such as trees or the grass in parks.

Cladosporium herbarium is the dominant fungal species in town and country, although present in higher concentration in the latter. *Penicillium Spp.* and *Aspergillus Spp.* on the other hand are relatively more common in urban areas (Davies *et al.*, 1963).

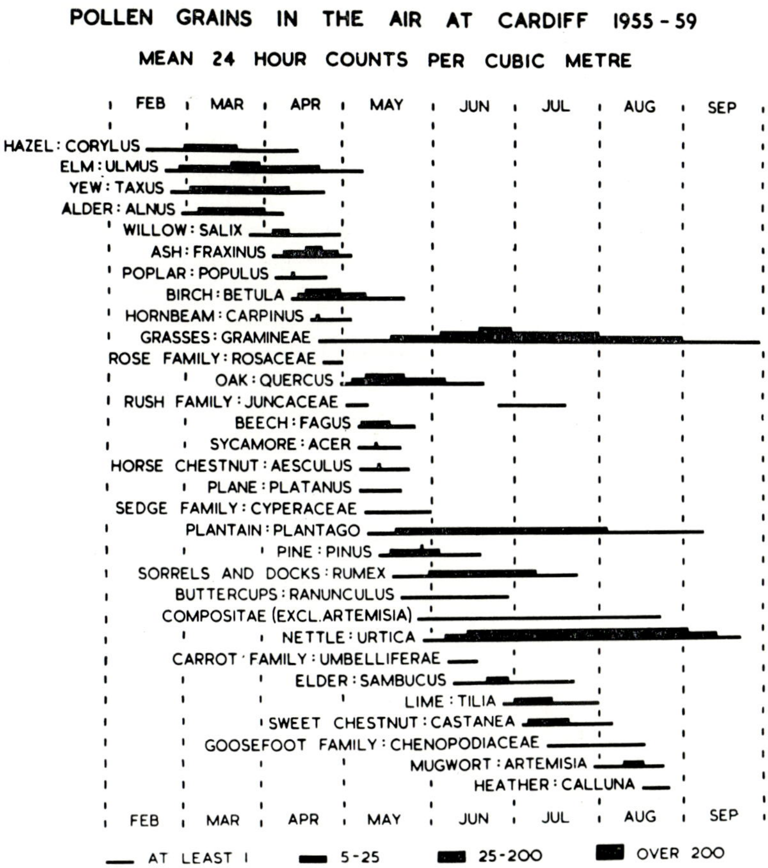

FIG. 1. (Reproduced from Acta. Allergol (1960) Suppl. VII.)

Diurnal Periodicity and the Effect of Weather

There are wide diurnal fluctuations in the particulate content of the air. For the most part these changes reflect the times at which the spores are released into the air and may be characteristic of each species. The controlling mechanism is probably the relative humidity (Hirst, 1953). The low humidity of warm sunny weather favours the release of grass pollen, *Alternaria* and *Cladosporium* during the daylight hours. The characteristic night spora is Sporobolomyces, ascospores and basidiospores. Their release is favoured by the high relative humidity during darkness. Very high concentrations in the air just before dawn may also be due to stable air conditions at this time which reduce turbulent mixing with cleaner air from higher altitudes (Gregory, 1961).

Rainfall has complex effects depending upon the size of the water drops and on the size of the particles. Pollen grains of about 30 μ diameter are rapidly washed out of the atmosphere, but the process is much less efficient with fungal spores below 4 μ in diameter. By contrast,

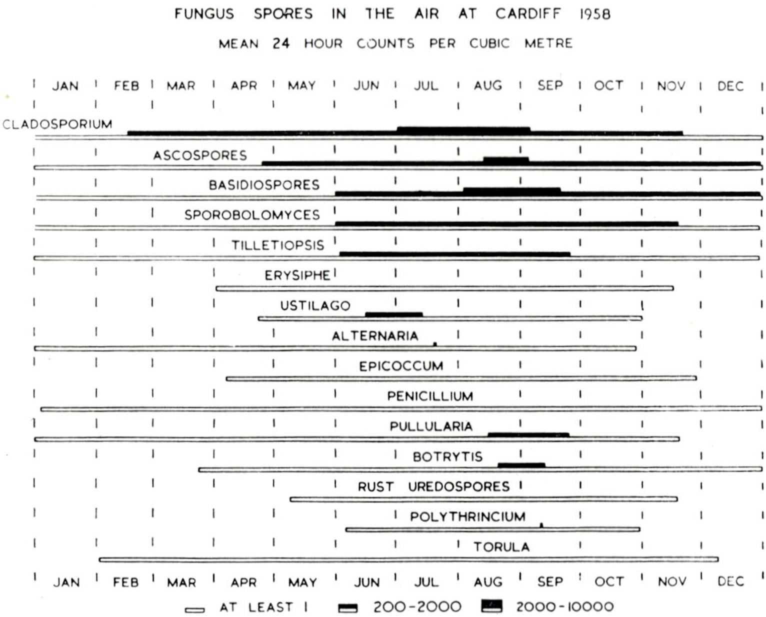

FIG. 2. (Reproduced from Acta. Allergol (1960) Suppl. VII.)

the falling droplets of water may lift spores off foliage and off the ground by a splash dispersal mechanism (Gregory *et al.*, 1959). The greater humidity also encourages the release of damp weather fungi such as *Sporobolomyces*.

The Effect of Altitude

Relief of allergic symptoms in some patients when residing at high altitudes has been noted for many years. Comparative studies in London and Davos (altitude 1,560 m) by Davies (1969) showed that the pollen and fungal spore content of the air at each situation was dominated by the local vegetation. London, having extensive parks and being near to the arable land of southern England, had relatively high grass pollen counts and also of ascospores such as *Leptosphaeria*, *Alternaria* and *Cladosporium* which are known to be associated with cereal crops. The basidiospore concentrations were higher at Davos, however, due to the proximity of extensive pine forests in which the fungi grow. The grass pollen counts at Davos were lower than those recorded in London although still high enough to cause symptoms in sensitive subjects. The absolute height of a region above sea level is probably of little importance, except for the beneficial effects of the low humidity in reducing mite infestation in houses in mountainous areas, which has already been noted.

Occupational Allergens

Unfamiliar allergens or unusual concentrations of familiar substances may be encountered in a patient's working environment. Many asthmatic subjects develop wheezing when exposed to any irritating dust or fumes, but this is due to reflex bronchoconstriction rather than to an allergic response. Some dusts from cotton, hemp, jute or flax may contain histamine releasing agents which are considered by some authors to cause asthmatic symptoms although this mechanism remains unproven.

True allergic asthma is not infrequent, however, although the association between the patient's symptoms and his exposure may be missed. Well-known occupational allergens include cat, dog or horse hair, grain dust, flour, gum acacia and some highly reactive gaseous compounds such as toluene di-isocyanate, formaldehyde, cyanuric chloride and ethylene diamine. Some metallic substances such as platinum, nickel, vanadium and tungsten in an aerosol form are known to cause asthma-like syndromes. Unlike natural allergens these occupational substances are not proteins but act as haptenes. The industrial causes of asthma are reviewed by Gandevia (1970). There is no information concerning the particle size of the allergens or of their concentrations in most instances. The isocyanate compounds appear to be able to cause severe symptoms in exceedingly small amounts.

High concentrations of some organic dusts cause an allergic response in the alveolar tissue of the lung. The dust must contain a high concentration of particles below about 7 μ in diameter which are thus able to penetrate to the alveoli. The known causes of this important group of diseases are rapidly expanding and they are reviewed in detail by Pepys (1969). Most occur in association with certain occupations, and the causative agent is often a fungal growth whose spores are of the appropriate size. The first to be recognized was Farmers' Lung due to *Micropolyspora faeni* (Pepys *et al.*, 1963). The spores are about 1 μ in diameter and may reach concentrations of 1600/cc of air in farm buildings (Lacey and Lacey, 1964). Fungi probably also cause a similar reaction in bagassosis, mushroom workers' lung, malt workers' lung (*Aspergillus clavatus* 3·5 μ), sequoiosis, maple bark disease (*Cryptostroma corticale* 5 $\mu \times 3 \mu$) and many more. Dust of mixed particle size but, presumably, containing sufficient material in the appropriate size range is associated with allergic alveolar disease in bird breeders, pituitary-snuff takers and those exposed to the wheat weavil, to bacterial enzymes used in the manufacture of washing powders, and possibly other vegetable dusts (Pepys *et al.*, 1964).

The rapid increase in knowledge of this important group of diseases during the last decade had been mainly through the use of skin tests, serology and allergic challenge techniques. The measurement of the size of the airborn particles and of their concentrations has been of less importance since exposure is inferred from the clinical history or by examination of the working site.

Deposition of Allergens in the Respiratory Tract

The behaviour of particles in the respiratory tract is described in Chapter 1. The general pattern of deposition of allergenic spores depends on the size of the particles, and natural organic aerosols are particularly interesting in this respect because of their remarkably uniform size. This is a situation rarely encountered with other dust clouds. So uniform are the spores of *Lycopodium* for example (about 30 μ in diameter) that they are often used as an experimental tool for the study of the aerodynamics of aerosols. This uniformity allows the site of deposition of the allergen in the lung to be stated with some precision. Much depends on whether the subject inhales through the nose or through the mouth. Mouth-breathing occurs during normal conversation, heavy exercise or when nasal obstruction is present as is often the case in allergic rhinitis. During nasal breathing all the pollen grains, and most of the larger fungal spores, are completely trapped in the nose. Smaller fungal spores, between 1 and 5 μ in diameter, may escape filtration and penetrate to the alveoli, although many are deposited on the surface of the upper airway as the tidal air carries them into the lung. During mouth breathing, however, fungal spores easily penetrate to the bronchial tree, and a fair proportion of pollen grains may also reach the second or third generation of airways.

The intensity of the antigen stimulus to the mucosa is closely related to the particle size. Spores of about one micron in diameter for example are probably distributed fairly uniformly throughout the lung so that the concentration of spores per unit area of lung surface is almost constant in all regions. Larger particles trapped in the nose result in a much more intense local exposure. This is well illustrated by comparing pollen grains with fungal spores. Frankland and Davies (1956) report that patients sensitive to grass pollen (diameter about 32 μ) develop symptoms when the airborne concentration reaches about $50/m^3$. Patients sensitive to *Cladosporium* spores (size about $10 \times 5\ \mu$) react when the concentration reaches $3{,}000/m^3$. The mass airborne concentration of pollen is only about twice that of the smaller fungal spores but those which are trapped in the nose are concentrated over a few square centimetres of mucosa. The fungal spores, on the other hand, are likely to be more uniformly distributed over a wide surface area in the bronchial tree.

The rate at which an insoluble particle is removed from the lung is also a function of the site of its deposition and hence of its size. Those penetrating to the alveoli are removed very slowly indeed and thus exert an antigenic stimulus out of all proportion to their total mass. Even in the case of allergens depositing on the ciliated epithelium those which penetrate nearer to the terminal bronchiole take longer to be expelled than those which are trapped in the trachea. The basidiospores, which, in Fig. 3, are shown to have a total mass second only to grass pollen, may thus exert a greater antigenic stimulus than the pollen simply because they are present on the mucosa for a longer time.

The optical size of a pollen grain or a fungal spore, as with all particles, may give only an approximate indication of its true aerodynamic size. The latter determines the pattern of its deposition in the lung. An extreme example is given by pollen of *Pinus sylvestris*. The individual grains are about 50 μ long by 35 μ wide, but the terminal velocity of the grain is equivalent to that of a 30 μ diameter sphere. The grains are thus quite capable of entering the nose with the tidal air but will be trapped at that point. In fact, most of the common pollens and spores appear to have particle sizes which are fairly close to their aerodynamic size as measured in the laboratory although there is only limited experimental information available, and it is possible that such unexplored factors as the humidity of the lungs may cause unexpected changes in the size of the particles.

Some fungi such as the *Aspergilli* and *Pencillia* are liberated in the form of chains containing a number of individual spores. Their rate of fall is a function of the diameter of the single spores and not of the length of the chain (Stober *et al.*, 1970). In sampling apparatuses, assuming that the chains are not broken in the airstreams, they would therefore be collected as if they were single spores. However, they tend to be deposited at a much higher point in the respiratory tract than their size would suggest. The details of this mechanism have been described in the case of asbestos fibres by Timbrell (1965).

The precise mechanism of asthma caused by house mites is unknown. Soysa and Jayawerdena (1945) found *Tyroglyphus* mites in the sputum of some of their patients with pulmonary eosinophilia. These insects are some 300 μ in diameter and, if they do reach the airways by inhalation, then this must be when the subject breathes with the mouth open.

Relative Importance of Different Allergens

It is not known why some airborne pollens and fungi cause symptoms and others do not. Nor is there any means of predicting this other than by the clinical assessment of each in turn. In general terms those pollens and moulds which are present in the greatest airborne concentrations for the longest period of time have been found to be the most common cause of symptoms. In this context Hyde and Adams (1960) pointed out that the mass concentration of the airborne material was the important measure, and not the number concentration irrespective of particle size.

Principal types of pollens and spores at Cardiff, 1958.

No.		Average mean daily concentration in spores per cubic metre	Size μ	Volume μ^3 (all approx.)	Mean daily volume μ^3/m^3 (all approx.)
1	Grasses	13.4	32(a)	17,164	229,998
2	Basidiospores	687	8 × 5(b)	157	107,859
3	Ascospores	368	10.5 × 5.5(c)	249.5	91,816
4	Cladosporium	446	10 × 4.5	159	70,914
5	Elm (Ulmus)	5.38	28	11,499	61,865
6	Birch (Betula)	3.69	22	5,578	20,583
7	Epicoccum	8.80	16	2,146	18,885
8	Alder (Alnus)	2.31	23	6,373	14,722
9	Beech (Fagus)	0.377	42	38,808	14,631
10	Alternaria	5.78	23.8 × 11.2(d)	2,346	13,560
11	Botrytis	27.5	11.3 × 7.3	473	13,008
12	Nettle (Urtica)	8.29	14	1,437	11,913
13	Oak (Quercus)	0.903	29	12,775	10,633
14	Hazel (Corylus)	1.25	24	7,241	9,051
15	Ash (Fraxinus)	1.62	22	5,578	9,036
16	Plantain (Plantago)	1.11	24	7,241	8,038
17	Tilletiopsis	177	9 × 2.5	44	7,788
18	Lime (Tilia)	0.467	31	15,605	7,288
19	Ustilago (Smut)	44.8	6.5	144	6,451
20	Sorrel & Dock (Rumex)	0.755	25	8,185	6,180
21	Sporobolomyces	295	3.5 × 2	11	3,245

Notes. (a) Timothy grass (*Phleum pratense*) taken as a typical 'wild' grass. (b) Average of 10 representative types. (c) Average of 10 representative types. (d) Average of 16 isolates of *A. tenuis* (Neergaard, Monograph of *Alternaria* and *Stemphylium* 1945).

FIG. 3. (Reproduced from Acta. Allergol (1960) Suppl. VII.)

The important allergens on a numerical basis and on a volume basis are shown in Fig. 3 (Hyde and Adams, 1960). The dominant position of grass pollen is evident and this is known to account for its role as the cause of the great majority of cases of pollenosis in Britain. *Cladosporium herbarium* is the fungal species associated with the highest average mass concentration and is the mould of most clinical significance (Frankland and Davies, 1965). The possible importance of the

Basidiomycetes is also obvious and attention was drawn to this by Gregory and Hirst (1952). Proven cases of allergy to the Basidiomycetes were reported by Herxheimer *et al.* (1969).

The chemical nature of the proteins in the particle and the rate of their release in the lung are other factors determining the allergenic potention of each species. Pine pollen, for example, is released in vast quantities over Northern regions but has rarely been known to cause symptoms (Newmark and Itkin, 1967).

The Relation Between Particle Size and the Allergic Response

The allergic manifestations depend on the concentration of antibody and antigen at a particular site and on the sensitivity of the tissues at that point to substances such as histamine. The differential deposition of inhaled antigen in various parts of the respiratory tract as a function of the size of the inhaled particles results in localized concentrations of antigen. The water soluble fraction of antigen may well be leached off the particles and obtain access to other regions of the lung or body through the blood stream so that inhaled allergens may cause eczema (Diamond, 1957; Tuft, 1960) or renal damage (Hardwick, 1959). Despite these reservations there is a general relationship in that large pollen grains which are trapped in the nose tend to cause rhinitis and conjunctivitis while smaller fungal spores, which can penetrate the nose, more typically cause asthma. Dusts containing a sufficient concentration of particles with aerodynamic diameters below about 5 or 6 microns are associated with the allergic alveolitis group of disorders. Many of these finer particles are also deposited in the upper respiratory tract, however, and it is not surprising that nasal symptoms, asthma and alveolitis may be caused by one and the same spore.

This overall picture has many exceptions. Most patients with severe hay fever of many years duration, eventually develop asthma, and some subjects with pollenosis have asthma without ever developing a reaction in the nose, where the grains are usually deposited. Fungal spores may be a potent cause of rhinitis without asthma, despite their ability to reach the bronchial tree. It is not known whether this discrepancy between the observed allergic response and the site of the deposition of the antigen is associated with an uneven distribution of antibody or of tissue sensitivity to the chemical products released by the antibody/antigen reaction. This variability causes difficulty over the question of diagnostic challenge techniques using extracts of antigen. A voluminous literature is now available on the relationship between the allergic response observed following the introduction of antigen into the skin and that following its direct application to the conjunctivae, nose or bronchi. Each may be positive when the others are negative, and the pattern may change in an individual patient whose clinical condition is apparently static. This change may possibly reflect a change in the distribution of antibody in the atopic subject, or of the non-specific reactivity of cells in different parts of the body. Some asthmatics are exquisitely sensitive to inhaled bronchoconstrictors, such as histamine or acetylcholine (Tiffenau, 1958), and this could be the main factor determining the degree of bronchoconstriction following challenge by inhaled antigen (Zuidema, 1969). The reactivity of an individual patient tends to increase with the level of natural exposure, and most pollen-sensitive subjects react more violently to bronchial challenge during the season than at other times (Feinberg and Steinberg, 1933). The increased sensitivity resulting from continuous antigen challenge is local in effect but may again be due to non-specific factors since the response to other allergens at that site is also increased (Connell, 1968).

In addition to the effects of particle size, there is some evidence that the pattern of the allergic response is an inherited characteristic (McKee, 1966) and that the tendency to develop rhinitis rather than asthma or the reverse is familial. Moreover, once the pattern becomes established, it tends to persist so that the same response develops whatever the site of deposition of further allergen. This is particularly evident in challenge tests. Subjects with hay-fever develop rhinitis, those with asthma wheeze (Hosen, 1965) and those with an allergic alveolitis develop the appropriate response. This occurs although each may be challenged with the same aerosol cloud. Such sprays usually contain a wide range of particle sizes, and the antigen presumably has access to most parts of the mucosal surface.

The total inhaled dose of antigen is easily controlled during such tests by measuring the length of exposure (Herxheimer, 1951) or by using solutions of different strengths (Makino, 1966). The use of particles of controlled sizes is much more difficult. Attempts to compare the effects of equivalent doses of antigen delivered to different regions of the lung by the use of particles of different size face the same problems as those relating to the therapeutic aerosols containing bronchodilators (see Chapter 9). Finer clouds are readily obtained by filtering out the larger droplets (Itkin *et al.*, 1963) but the value of doing this remains to be established. Since very soluble compounds are absorbed from the surface of the mucosa at about the same speed as if given by intravenous injection, the particle size of liquid aerosols and hence the site of their deposition may be of little importance. It is certainly unlikely that the response will be identical to that following the inhalation of actual fungal spores, or of pollen grains, which release their antigen relatively slowly and which cause it to be concentrated at a particular site in the lung. The choice of aerosols of a defined particle size might be particularly important in desensitization by the inhalation method. If this is shown to have advantages over parenteral administration in some instance, then the antigen should presumably be deposited at the same site in the lung as that during natural exposure.

Avoiding the Allergen

Such simple measures as remaining indoors and closing the windows when the pollen count is high, are effective and well known to patients. The pollen count can be further reduced indoors by means of air filtration systems throughout the house or in particular rooms. Small nasal filters and shielded spectacles may benefit sensitive subjects and enable them to move freely outside the home (Little, 1968). Moving to another district, or country, may produce benefit but, of course, atopic patients are likely to become sensitive to further allergens in the new environment. Temporary residence in an allergen-reduced region may be of real benefit to severely disabled patients, particularly children. Unfortunately, such individuals may occasionally be more than usually sensitive on returning to their customary home (Storm van Leeuwen, 1924).

If a local cause can be identified, then it must obviously be dealt with by appropriate means. This is not always easy where a man's employment is concerned. The use of well-fitting respirators may be helpful in situations where exposure is unlikely to be continuous. There is no doubt that such methods may enable farmers to continue work without ill effects, despite further exposure to mouldy hay (Gourley and Braidwood, 1971).

It is difficult to prove that a general reduction in the amount of dust in the house is of benefit (Report Brit. Tub. Assoc., 1968) although this is part of the accepted management of asthmatics sensitive to house dust. The possibility that such sensitivity is dominated by house mites has permitted a more rational approach. Methods of reducing the mite population by the cleaning of mattresses and bed linen are described by Maunsell (1970). Although sealing of the mattress in an airtight cover is unnecessary, it should be vacuumed weekly, and clothing and blankets should be washed frequently. The use of insecticides cannot be considered to be desirable as yet, but it may be possible to reduce the mite population by keeping the room dry and by lowering the relative humidity yet further by means of central heating. Very sparse mite populations appear to be present in hospital wards. This is probably due to the complete and frequent changes of bed linen and may explain the improvement in the symptoms of some asthmatics which has been so often noted following their admission to hospital.

References

Adams, K. F. and Hyde, H. A. (1965), "Pollen Grains and Fungal Spores Indoors and Out at Cardiff." *J. Palynol.*, **1**, 67.

Blackley, C. H. (1873), *Experimental Researches on the Causes and Nature of Catarrhus Aestivus* (*Hay-fever or Hay-asthma*). Baillière Tindall & Co.

British Tuberculosis Association (1968), "Report of Research Committee on Treatment of House Dust Allergy." *Brit. Med. J.*, **2**, 774.

Connell, J. T. (1968), "Quantitative Intranasal Pollen Challenge." *J. Allergy*, **41,** 123.
Cunnington, A. M. and Gregory, P. H. (1968), "Mites in Bedroom Air." *Nature, Lond.*, **217,** 1271.
Davies, R. R. (1965), "Pollen and Fungal Spores in City Atmosphere." *Acta Allerg.*, **20,** 508.
Davies, R. R. (1969), "Aerobiology and the Relief of Asthma in an Alpine Valley." *Acta Allerg.*, **24,** 377.
Davies, R. R., Derry, M. J. and Newton, L. M. (1963), "A Comparison Between the Summer and Autumn Air-spores at London and Liverpool." *Acta Allerg.*, **18,** 131.
Dekker, H. (1928), "Asthma und Milben." *Münch med. Wschr.*, **75,** 515.
Diamond, H. E. (1957), "Atopic Dermatitis due to Inhalation." *N.Y. State J. Med.*, **57,** 754.
Feinberg, S. M. and Steinberg, M. G. (1933), "Studies in Pollen Potency." *J. Allergy*, **5,** 19.
Floyer, Sir John (1698), "A Treatise on the Asthma."
Frankland, A. W. and Davies, R. R. (1965), "Allergie aux spores de moississures en Angleterre." *Le Poumon et le Cocur*, *I*, 11.
Frankland, A. W., McEwan, L. M. and Feinberg, J. G. (1970), "Skin Reactions to Dust and Mites." *Int. Arch. Allergy*, **37,** 351.
Gandevia, B. (1970), "Occupational Asthma." *Med. J. Aust.*, **2,** 332.
Gourley, G. A. and Braidwood, G. D. (1971), "The Use of Respirators in the Prevention of Recurrence of Farmers' Lung." *Trans. Soc. Occ. Med.* (In press.)
Gregory, P. H. (1961), *Microbiology of the Atmosphere*. London: Hill.
Gregory, P. H. and Hirst, J. M. (1952), "Possible Role of Basidiospores as Air-borne Allergens." *Nature, Lond.*, **170,** 414.
Gregory, P. H., Guthrie, E. J. and Bunce, M. E. (1958), "Experiments on the Splash Dispersal of Fungus Spores." *J. gen. Microbiol.*, **29,** 328.
Hamilton, E. D. (1959), "Studies on the Air Spora." *Acta Allerg.*, **13,** 143.
Hardwick, J. (1959), "Nephrotic Syndrome with Pollen Hypersensitivity." *Lancet*, **i,** 500.
Harrington, J. B. (1959), "High Efficiency Pollen Samplers for Use in Clinical Allergy." *J. Allergy*, **30,** 357.
Herxheimer, H. (1951), "Induced Asthma in Man." *Lancet*, **1,** 1337.
Herxheimer, H., Hyde, H. A. and Williams, D. A. (1969), "Allergic Asthma Caused by Basidiospores. *Lancet*, **ii,** 13.
Hirst, J. M. (1952), "An Automatic Volumetric Spore Trap." *Ann. Appl. Biol.*, **39,** 257.
Hirst, J. M. (1953), "Changes in Atmospheric Spore Content: Diurnal Periodicity and the Effects of Weather." *Trans. Br. Mycol. Soc.*, **36,** 375.
Hosen, H. (1965), "Provocative Nasal Tests for Diagnosis of Inhalant Allergens." *Ann. Allergy*, **23,** 497.
Hyde, H. A. (1952), "Grass Pollen and Hay Fever in Great Britain." *Acta Allerg.*, **57,** 98.
Hyde, H. A. (1956), "Tree Pollens in Great Britain." *Acta Allerg.*, **10,** 224.
Hyde, H. A. (1959), " 'Weed' Pollen in Great Britain." *Acta Allerg.*, **13,** 186.
Hyde, H. A. (1969), "Aeropalynology in Britain—an Outline." *New Phytol.*, **68,** 579.
Hyde, H. A. and Adams, K. F. (1960), "Airborne Allergens at Cardiff 1942–59." *Acta Allerg.* (Suppl. VII), 159.
Itkin, I. H., Anend, S., Yau, M. and Middlebrooke, E. (1963), "Quantitative Inhalation Challenge in Allergic Asthma." *J. Allergy*, **34,** 97.
Kirkman, W. P. (1862), "Der typische Fruhsommer Katarrh." In *Pheobus, P.*, p. 137.
Lacey, J. and Lacey, M. E. (1964), "Spore Concentrations in the Air of Farm Buildings." *Trans. Brit. Mycol. Soc.*, **47,** 547.
Little, E. C. S. (1968), "Keeping Pollen at Bay." *Lancet*, **2,** 512.

McKee, W. D. (1966), "The Incidence and Familial Occurrence of Allergy." *J. Allergy*, **38**, 226.

Makino, S. (1966), "Clinical Significance of Bronchial Sensitivity to Acetylcholine and Histamine in Bronchial Asthma." *J. Allergy*, **38**, 127.

Maunsell, K. (1952), "Airborne Fungal Spores Before and After Raising Dust." *Int. Arch. Allergy appl. Immun.*, **3**, 93.

Maunsell, K. (1970), "Mite Asthma: Cause and Management." *Practitioner*, **205**, 779.

Maunsell, K., Wraith, D. G. and Cunnington, A. M. (1968), "Mites and House Dust Allergy in Bronchial Asthma." *Lancet*, **1**, 1267.

Newmark, F. M. and Itkin, I. H. (1967), "Asthma due to Pine Pollen." *Ann. Allergy*, **25**, 251.

Pepys, J. (1969), *Hypersensitivity Diseases of the Lungs due to Fungi.* Basel and New York: Karger.

Pepys, J., Jenkins, P. A., Festenstein, G. N., Gregory, P. H., Lacey, M. and Skinner, F. A. (1963). "Farmers' Lung: Thermophilic Actinomycetes as a Source of 'Farmers' Lung Hay' Antigen." *Lancet*, **ii**, 607.

Pepys, J., Longbottom, J. L. and Jenkins, P. A. (1964), "Vegetable Dust Pneumoconiosis. Immunological Responses to Vegetable Dusts and Their Flora." *Amer. Rev. resp. Dis.*, **89**, 842.

Richards, M. (1954), "Atmospheric Mould Spores In and Out of Doors." *J. Allergy*, **25**, 429.

Soysa, E. and Jayawardena, M. D. S. (1945), "Pulmonary Acariasis. A Possible Cause of Asthma." *Brit. Med. J.*, **1**, 1.

Spieksma, F. T. M. (1967), *The House-dust Mite Dermatophagoides Pteronysinus* (Trouessart, 1897). Leiden: Proefschrift.

Stöber, W., Flachsbart, H. and Hochrainer, D. (1970), "The Aerodynamic Diameter of Latex Aggregates and Asbestos Fibres." *Staub-Reinhalt*, **30**, 1.

Storm van Leeuwen, W. (1924), "Bronchial Asthma in Relation to Climate." *Proc. R. Soc. Med.*, **17** (Sect. Therap. and Pharmacol.), 19.

Thommen, A. A. (1931), "Etiology of Hay-fever: Studies in Hay-fever." *N.Y. State J. Med.*, **30**, 437.

Tiffenau, R. (1958), "Hypersensibilities cholinergo-histaminique-pulmonaire de l'asthmatique." *Acta Allergol.*, Suppl. V, **18**, 198.

Timbrell, V. (1965), "The Inhalation of Fibrous Dusts." *Annals of the New York Acad. of Sci.*, **132**, 255.

Tuft, L. (1960), "Studies in Atopic Dermatitis." *J. Allergy*, **31**, 1.

Voorhorst, R., Spieksma–Boezeman, M. I., Spieksma, F. T. (1964), *Allergie Asthma*, **10**, 329.

Zuidema, P. (1969), "Value of Inhalation Tests in Bronchial Asthma." *Respiration*, **26** (Suppl.), 141.

Chapter 5

Byssinosis

R. S. F. Schilling

Introduction

The asthmatic complaints of carders of hemp and flax were first described by Bernadino Ramazzini (1713), the Italian physician and pioneer of industrial medicine. Later, Patissier (1822) in France, wrote of a similar disease affecting cotton workers. The disease, now called byssinosis (derived from *βυσσος* meaning linen or fine flax) is caused by the dust emitted in processing cotton, flax and soft hemp (cannabis sativa). Byssinosis occurs principally among workers cleaning and preparing fibres for spinning. It is characterized by chest tightness and breathlessness at work after the weekend break or other absence. In the later stages, which usually develop after many years of exposure to dust, the worker is severely disabled with symptoms which cannot be distinguished from those of chronic bronchitis and emphysema.

Cotton

In cotton manufacture, byssinosis may affect workers in ginneries where seeds are removed from the picked cotton bolls, in pressing the cotton into bales and in the mixing and card rooms where the fibres are cleaned and combed. The introduction of mechanical picking has increased the contamination of cotton with plant debris and the general speeding up of all processes has raised dust concentrations in work rooms with the result that the disease now occurs in spinning and winding (Mekky, Roach and Schilling, 1967).

Flax

Among flax workers, byssinosis occurs in preparatory processes in factories making linen (Carey, Elwood, McAuley, Merrett and Pemberton, 1965). It has been found among the inhabitants of an Egyptian village where flax is processed in the homes (El Batawi and Hussein, 1964). Both flax workers and members of their family were affected by the dust generated in and around their houses. Young children able to describe their symptoms were also found to suffer from the disease.

Soft Hemp

An asthma-like complaint called cannabosis was described by Barbero and Flores (1944) in Spanish workers making ropes and twines from soft hemp (Cannabis Sativa). It has since proved to be indistinguishable from the byssinosis of cotton and flax workers (Bouhuys, Barbero, Lindell, Roach and Schilling, 1967). More recently, byssinosis has been described among workers in Jugoslavia processing soft hemp (Valić, Žuškin, Walford, Keršić and Pauković, 1968).

Jute and other Vegetable Dusts

Jute emits a great deal of dust during processing, but it does not appear to cause byssinosis although it may cause workers to suffer unduly from chronic respiratory disease (Schilling, 1956). Recent surveys indicate that in spite of high dust exposure in processing vegetable fibres like St. Helena Hemp, manila and sisal, there is no specific hazard of byssinosis although their dusts may cause persistent cough and expectoration, with a fall in the ventilatory capacity of the lungs during the work shift (Munt, Gauvain, Walford and Schilling, 1965; McKerrow, Gilson, Schilling and Skidmore, 1965). The effects from exposure to high concentrations of jute, manila, St. Helena Hemp and sisal are probably mechanical in origin and caused by rapid reflex response with bronchoconstriction; it is essentially a different response to that produced by the dusts which cause byssinosis.

In the manufacture of man-made fibres there is no risk of byssinosis (Tiller and Schilling, 1958). The production of cotton is rising about twice as fast as man-made fibres due to rapid expansion in developing countries. The use of flax is diminishing but although man-made fibres are replacing hemp in the manufacture of nets, there is no decrease in hemp production. Thus, the substitution of natural by man-made fibres is unlikely to eliminate the problem of byssinosis. The building of new textile factories in developing countries to process the natural fibres which are grown in abundance is an important part of their economic expansion (Gilson, 1968).

Symptomatology and Diagnosis

In the early stages of the disease there are characteristic symptoms of chest tightness on the first day of work after the weekend. In Western countries this occurs on Mondays and may develop during the first year of exposure. The feeling of tightness or difficulty in breathing usually comes on towards the end of the shift and disappears shortly after leaving the workplace. On Tuesdays, the worker has no symptoms. As the disease progresses, the chest tightness and breathlessness worsens and extends to Tuesdays and then to other days. At this stage, symptoms still improve as the week goes on. Eventually, the worker may become severely affected on every working day with permanent and severe effort intolerance and a markedly impaired ventilatory capacity which is not improved by him giving up his dusty occupation.

In its final stages, byssinosis cannot be distinguished from non-occupational chronic bronchitis and emphysema except for the past history of chest tightness characteristically worse at the beginning of the working week. The textile worker with byssinosis often forgets his early symptoms and is diagnosed as suffering from non-occupational chronic respiratory disease. Chest X-rays do not show changes specific for byssinosis, nor has any specific pathology been identified in the lungs of workers who have died of this disease. The X-ray or pathological changes in the lungs are those found in chronic bronchitis and emphysema.

There are two methods or assessing the prevalence and severity of byssinosis and of aiding diagnosis. Respiratory symptoms may be graded by using a standardized questionnaire. Ventilatory capacity may be measured and graded before and after work, preferably on a Monday before the worker has become acclimatized to the dust.

Questionnaire

Respiratory symptoms, past history of chest disease, smoking habits and occupational histories are recorded using a standard questionnaire on respiratory symptoms (Lammers, Schilling and Walford, 1964; British Occupational Hygiene Society, 1971). This questionnaire has been extensively used in many countries and has proved a valuable aid to diagnosis. The symptoms of byssinosis are graded as follows:

Grade 0	No symptoms of byssinosis
Grade $\frac{1}{2}$	Occasional chest tightness on the first day of the working week
Grade 1	Chest tightness on every first day of the working week
Grade 2	Chest tightness on the first and other days of the working week
Grade 3	Grade 2 symptoms accompanied by evidence of permanent incapacity from diminished effort tolerance and/or reduced ventilatory capacity

Ventilatory function tests. Exposure to the dusts of cotton, flax and soft hemp causes both temporary and permanent changes in ventilatory capacity. The most commonly used test is the Forced Expiratory Volume over 1·0 second ($FEV_{1\cdot0}$). Measured on a Monday at the beginning and end of the shift, it provides additional evidence of the byssinosis hazard and helps to identify those workers who are susceptible to the dust. In practice, those workers with symptoms of byssinosis have significantly greater falls in ventilatory capacity during the work shift than those without symptoms.

The $FEV_{1\cdot0}$ measured before dust exposure or while the subject is absent from work also provides evidence of the permanent effects of dust exposure and is important in assessing his disability and deciding whether a worker should be advised to change his occupation.

A grading of acute and permanent changes in ventilatory capacity is as follows (Bouhuys, Gilson and Schilling, 1970)—

- F0 No demonstrable acute effect of the dust on ventilatory capacity; no evidence of chronic ventilatory impairment
- F½ Slight acute effect of dust on ventilatory capacity; no evidence of chronic ventilatory impairment
- F1 Definite acute effect of dust on ventilatory capacity; no evidence of chronic ventilatory impairment
- F2 Evidence of a slight to moderate irreversible impairment of ventilatory capacity
- F3 Evidence of a moderate to severe irreversible impairment of ventilatory capacity

The acute effect is measured by the fall in $FEV_{1\cdot 0}$ from the beginning to the end of the work shift on the first working day of the week, and is classified thus:

Less than 0·06 litres	no acute effect
0·06–0·20 litres	slight acute effect
Over 0·20 litres	definite acute effect

Chronic ventilatory impairment may be measured by the $FEV_{1\cdot 0}$ in the absence of exposure for 2 days or more in relation to the $FEV_{1\cdot 0}$ expected for a normal person of the same race, age and height (Cotes, 1968).

The results may be classified as follows:

Over 80% of predicted	no chronic ventilatory impairment
60–80% of predicted	moderate chronic ventilatory impairment
Less than 60% of predicted	severe chronic ventilatory impairment

Both the acute and the more permanent effects of cotton dust exposure on ventilatory capacity are well illustrated by the results of a study of male cotton workers in Holland (Walford, Lammers and Schilling, 1966). The cotton workers with byssinosis have significantly lower ventilatory capacities at the beginning of the shift than workers without symptoms. They also showed a marked fall in ventilatory capacity during the shift whereas workers without symptoms show changes compatible with the normal diurnal rhythms of lung function very similar to those of non-textile workers (Figure 1).

These results from surveys of men actively employed in cotton mills do not include those who left the industry because of respiratory disability. A survey of active and retired hemp workers and other workers reveals the extent of the permanent disability which can occur among the older men (Bouhuys, Barbero, Schilling and van de Woestigne, 1969). In the age group 50–69 years hemp workers had a significantly higher proportion of men with reduced ventilatory capacity than those who had never worked in hemp.

Nearly a third of the hemp workers of this age had more than a 50% reduction in $FEV_{1 \cdot 0}$, compared with expected values. The corresponding figure among the control subjects was 4% (Table 1).

Table 1

Actual $FEV_{1 \cdot 0}$*s* vs. *expected values in control subjects and hemp workers*

		$FEV_{1 \cdot 0}$			
Age 20–39	*Number of men*	<80% *of expected value**		<50% *of expected value**	
		No.	%	*No.*	%
Hemp workers	43	2	5	0	0
Controls	75	3	4	0	0
Age 40–49					
Hemp Workers	27	4	15	0	0
Controls	83	6	7	2	2
Age 50–69					
Hemp workers	146	89	61†	45	31†
Controls	89	21	24	4	4·5

* Expected values from Veterans Administration nomogram (Boren, Kory and Syner, 1966).

† $p < 0{\cdot}005$.

Effort Intolerance

The grading of effort intolerance is another means of assessing incapacity and is as follows:

Grade 1 *Normal*—not troubled by shortness of breath when hurrying on the level or walking up a slight gradient.

Grade 2 *Slight*—troubled by shortness of breath when hurrying on the level or walking up a slight gradient.

Grade 3 *Moderate*—short of breath walking with other people at an ordinary pace on the level.

Grade 4 *Severe*—having to stop for breath when walking at own pace on the level.

Although the grading of effort intolerance is a crude measure of disability, it indicates the serious nature of the respiratory disease

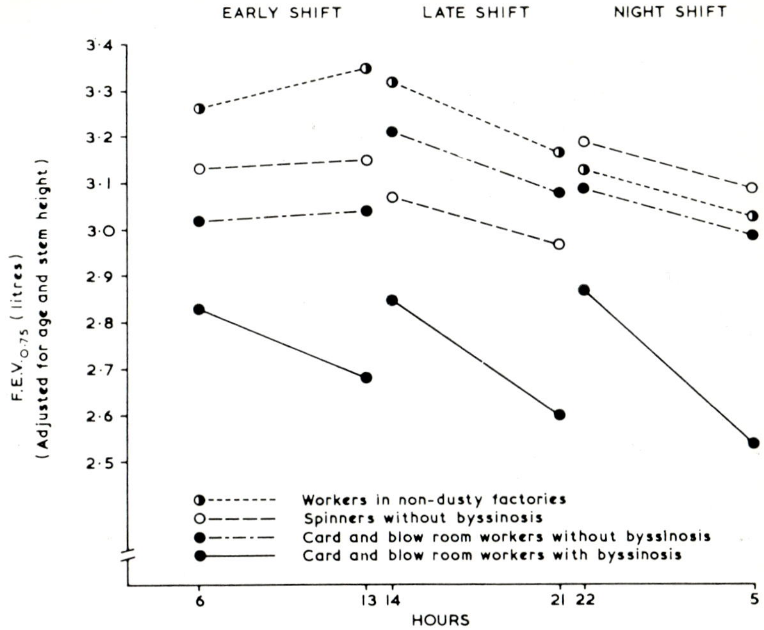

FIG. 1. Mean change in $FEV_{0\cdot 75}$ during shifts for cotton workers with and without byssinosis and workers in non-dusty factories.

among cotton workers spinning the coarse cotton which is reputedly very dusty (Schilling, 1962). The dyspnoea grading of 186 cotton workers are compared with those of 88 workers in an engineering factory in the same area. None of the engineers, but 10% of the cotton workers complained of moderate or severe dyspnoea when not at work (Table 2).

Table 2

Effort intolerance in 186 cotton and 88 other workers in an English cotton town

Effort intolerance at weekends	*Cotton workers* %	*Other workers* %
Normal (I)	66	90
Slight (II)	24	10
Moderate (III)	8	0
Severe (IV)	2	0

Pathogenesis

Until recently, physicians, particularly those in hospitals or chest clinics, seeing only the disabled workers presenting symptoms of chronic bronchitis, have been reluctant to recognize byssinosis as an occupational disease. They find its odd clinical history and lack of specific radiographic or pathological changes in the lungs unconvincing. Instead, men have been diagnosed as suffering from non-specific chronic respiratory disease. Pulmonary function tests used in epidemiological surveys of cotton workers provided additional and objective evidence that byssinosis is a separate disease and unlike the chronic bronchitis prevalent in the mill towns of Lancashire. The initial symptoms of chest tightness on Mondays are accompanied by a temporary reduction in ventilatory function and an increase in airways resistance. These changes, which are greater in workers with symptoms of byssinosis, are reversed by bronchodilatory drugs (McKerrow, McDermott, Gilson and Schilling, 1958; Bouhuys, Heaphy, Schilling and Welborn, 1967).

Workers with byssinosis also have a lower average ventilatory capacity, after adjusting for age and height, than those without the disease even when they are not exposed to dust. Bronchodilator drugs have relatively little effect particularly on older workers, indicating that they have irreversible changes in ventilatory capacity.

A reasonable hypothesis is that acute changes in ventilatory capacity eventually lead to an irreversible loss of function and that these changes are not primarily caused by mechanical constriction but by pharmacologically active substances producing bronchoconstriction. There is some conflict of opinion as to the mechanism by which inhaled dust has its acute effect on pulmonary ventilation. There are, for example, a number of agents in cotton dust which could cause a narrowing of the bronchioles by muscle constriction and/or oedema of the mucosa. They are histamine, antigenic and non-antigenic histamine releasing factors and 5-hydroxytryptamine; histamine itself and 5-hydroxytryptamine are usually present in such small quantities that they are unlikely to be important.

Massoud and Taylor (1964) have described an antibody directed against an antigen present in the cotton plant. The antigen is considered to be a polymer of leucocyanidin with smaller amounts of leucodelphinidin (Taylor, Massoud and Lucas, 1971). The titre of this antibody is higher in cardroom workers than in normal people and is highest in those who have byssinosis. The cotton plant antigen in its pure state, showed no significant toxic effects on mice and rats and no histamine-like or histamine-releasing activity. Bronchial challenge of human volunteers with the antigen in saline aerosol, produced symptoms similar to the Monday tightness in men with byssinosis, but not in normal or in non-byssinotic card-room workers. No changes were detected in $FEV_{1 \cdot 0}$ after challenge in subjects either with or without byssinosis. On the other hand, Bouhuys (1966) and his co-workers have produced evidence in favour of a non-antigenic histamine releasing agent being the cause of byssinosis.

Extracts of cotton, flax and hemp dust when incubated with human lung tissue in vitro, cause histamine release (Nicholls, Nicholls and Bouhuys, 1966). Recent work suggests that the bronchoconstriction agent in cotton dust may be methyl piperonylate (Hitchcock, Piscitelli and Bouhuys, 1971). Aqueous extracts of cotton dust and of the bracts from the cotton plant, cause chest tightness in healthy subjects at first exposure and a temporary reduction in ventilatory capacity. These extracts have a similar but more pronounced effect on the worker with symptoms of byssinosis. A second exposure to cotton dust extract 24 hours after the first, produces less effect. The relatively slow onset of symptoms, particularly in the early stages of the disease, is not characteristic of an asthma in persons who have become sensitized to an antigen; and since a large proportion of persons exposed have symptoms of byssinosis it seems unlikely that it is an allergic disease. The presence of a broncho-constricting agent in cotton flax or hemp dust causing non-antigenic release of histamine could explain the typical Monday symptoms. Most of the histamine available in lung tissue is released and acts upon the airways on the first working day, but little or no histamine is again available for release until the subject has been absent from work.

This, however, does not explain why the patient with severe byssinosis eventually becomes disabled with persistent symptoms which have a fairly rapid onset after exposure to dust. It is possible that both non-antigenic and antigenic histamine release agents may be aetiologically important in this complex disease.

Other Aetiological Factors

The relationship between cigarette smoking and non-specific chronic respiratory disease is well established—smoking is widely accepted as a major cause of chronic bronchitis. There is evidence from surveys of textile workers that byssinosis symptoms are more prevalent among smokers than among non-smokers (Schilling, 1964)—many sufferers from byssinosis are obliged to give up smoking because it aggravates the unpleasant effects of the dust. The survey of active and retired hemp workers (Bouhuys *et al.*, 1969) revealed an unexpected finding; unlike the control subjects the moderate to heavy smokers had significantly higher $FEV_{1.0}$s than the non- or light smokers among men aged 50–69. The ex-smokers show the lowest $FEV_{1.0}$s of all (Fig. 2). The most likely explanation is that the hemp workers who are susceptible to the dust cut down or give up smoking because they have relatively low $FEV_{1.0}$s. Those who are less susceptible to hemp dust remain healthy and continue to smoke. This suggests that cigarette smoking may be less deleterious than hemp dust, at least as far as the development of chronic respiratory symptoms and decreased ventilatory capacity is concerned.

When disabling byssinosis was regarded as a relatively uncommon disease confined to the Lancashire cotton industry, the adverse environment of the mill towns, particularly their polluted atmosphere, was considered a vital factor in causing disability (British Medical Journal, 1962). The world wide prevalence of byssinosis discounts this hypothesis. Few climates could be balmier or less polluted than the Nile Delta or the Carolinas in the United States where disabling byssinosis occurs (El Batawi, Schilling, Valić and Walford, 1964; Bouhuys, Heaphy, Schilling and Welborn, 1967).

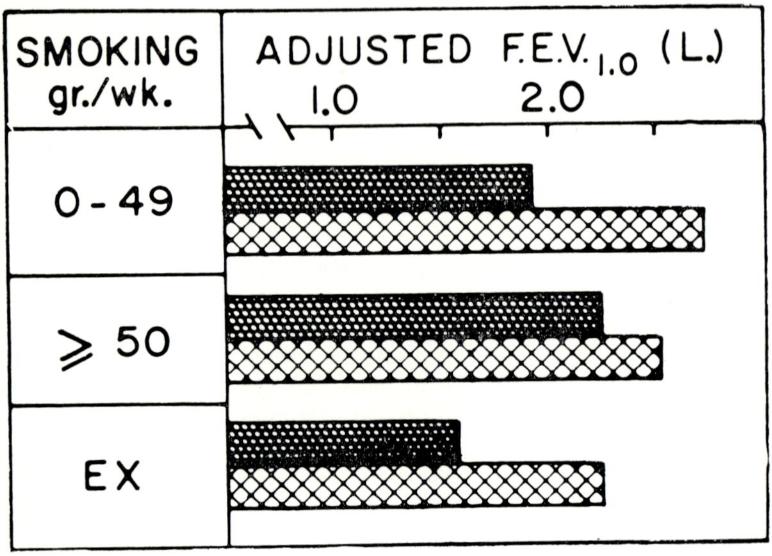

FIG. 2. Mean adjusted $FEV_{1\cdot0}$ in hempworkers (⁙) and control subjects (▩) aged 50–69 years in different smoking categories. Differences between hemp workers and controls are significant in all 3 categories ($p <$ 0·025 to $p <$ 0·005). Other significance tests:

	Controls	*Hemp workers*
0–49 *vs.* ≥ 50	$p <$ 0·05	$p <$ 0·025
0–49 *vs.* Ex	$p <$ 0·01	NS
50 *vs.* Ex	NS	$p <$ 0·005

0–49 and ≥50 indicate present smoking in grams/week.
Ex—ex-smokers.

A survey of English and Dutch mills spinning the same types of cotton revealed similar prevalences of byssinosis in both countries but a higher prevalence of chronic bronchitis among the English (Lammers, Schilling and Walford, 1967). Atmospheric pollution was much higher in the English towns and there was evidence among the workers with byssinosis that the English were more disabled than the Dutch. It seems likely that byssinosis is a more disabling disease in countries where chronic bronchitis is prevalent (Schilling, Vigliani, Lammers, Valić and Gilson, 1963).

Hygiene Standards

The prevalence of byssinosis symptoms is closely related to dust exposure as shown in Fig. 3 which is based on data from an epidemiological survey of 458 cotton workers by Roach and Schilling (1960). There is a point on the dose response curve at which no one is affected with Grade 1 symptoms.

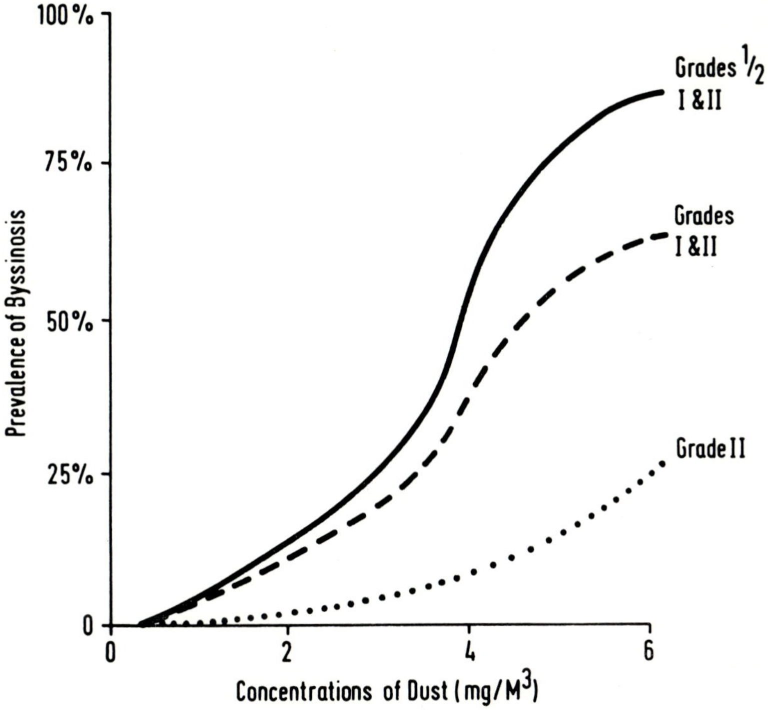

FIG. 3. Response to cotton dust exposure.

From these results the American Conference of Governmental Industrial Hygienists recommended as Threshold Limit Value (TLV) of 1 mg/M^3 total dust for cotton. Further investigations confirmed that where dust levels were near 1 mg/M^3 in workrooms without any modern exhaust ventilation system there was a very low prevalence of byssinosis (Mekky *et al.*, 1967; Smith, Coles, Schilling and Walford, 1969). The fall in ventilatory capacity during the shift is another way of measuring response to dust of a group of workers. In a survey of Egyptian card rooms workers processing high quality cotton acute changes in the indirect maximum breathing capacity showed a close correlation with dust exposure and prevalence of byssinosis symptoms (El Batawi, Schilling, Valić and Walford, 1964) (Fig. 4).

Recent studies in mills with modern air conditioning and other devices for removal of dust, have shown a higher response for the same weight of dust (Molyneux and Tombleson, 1970; Žuškin, Wolfson, Harpel, Welborn and Bouhuys, 1969). This is probably because the larger particles had been removed. There is good evidence that it is the finer dust particles (e.g. under 7 μ equivalent diameter) which produce the acute changes in respiratory function and so cause respiratory disability (McKerrow, Roach, Gilson and Schilling, 1962). Hygiene Standards have recently been reviewed by the British Occupational

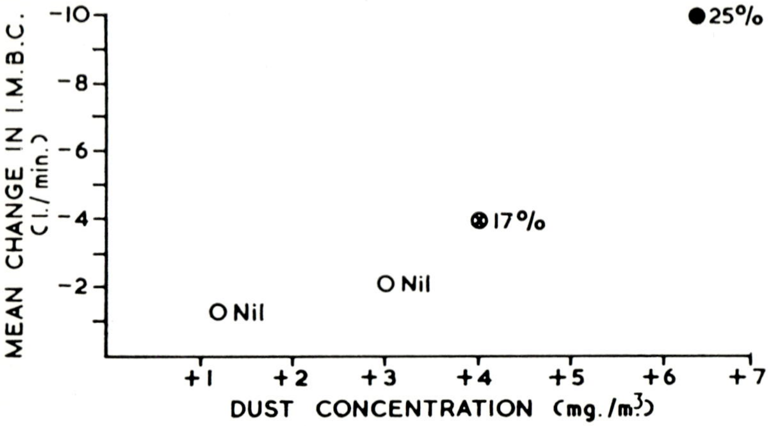

FIG. 4. Dust concentrations (mg/m³) and changes in indirect maximum breathing capacity (litres/min) in card rooms spinning fine cotton. The percentage figures refer to the prevalence of Byssinosis in the four card rooms in which the measurements were made.

Hygiene Society (1971). The recommended TLV is a maximum average concentration of 0·5 mg/M³ less fly. This excludes large particles which would be caught by a 2 mm wire mesh gauze or which would not enter a vertical elutriator designed to accept 50% of unit density spheres 30 μ in diameter. At these levels, the risk of workers being permanently affected by the dust would be very low. Where dust concentrations exceed this level medical surveillance is necessary (see below).

Prevention

Substitution of natural by man-made fibres offers no immediate solution to the problem of byssinosis. In the foreseeable future prevention will depend primarily on better dust control but there is no evidence that any one of the engineering devices used to suppress dust is entirely successful, as it is the less harmful coarse dust which is mostly removed by such devices. With the general speeding up of processes in the manufacture of cotton, dust is now being produced by other machines than carding engines. This makes the need for engineering control more widespread and more costly.

As many new plants are being installed in developing countries, where the industry plays an important part in the economy, there is an opportunity for making dust control an integral part of the design of all new textile equipment. General housekeeping in which the usual sweeping up is replaced by vacuum cleaning is essential whatever exhaust systems and enclosures are applied. Systematic dust sampling which is rarely done in factories processing natural fibres, is an essential part of dust control. Byssinosis seldom occurs in mills producing medical cotton which is treated with sodium hydroxide and bleached. As the pharmacologically active substances are water soluble, the possibility of washing cotton to remove harmful substances before processing should be considered. Similarly, the plant debris might be removed by some mechanical method before the cotton is ginned. At present, the plant debris which contains the active agent is crushed and rolled with the fibres and then has to be taken out when the fibres are mixed and carded. If either of these methods were practicable the problem of byssinosis in the cotton industry would be virtually solved.

Medical Surveillance

Until the harmful dust can be completely removed from workrooms, medical surveillance will be an important adjunct to environmental control. It should include initial and periodical examination (British Occupational Hygiene Society, 1971).

The initial medical examination aims to exclude from those parts of the process known to cause byssinosis, persons who have a history of atopic asthma, chronic non-specific lung disease, tuberculosis or any specific lung disease in which respiratory disability is a feature in the earlier stages. Those who are to be exposed to dust should be discouraged from smoking and non-smokers should be preferred for such jobs.

The periodic medical examination has two functions. It detects workers who are susceptible to dust among byssinosis; they can be moved to less dusty occupations before they develop any substantial disability. Secondly, the systematic examination of groups of workers is a valuable method of checking the adequacy of dust control and detecting those occupations where more control is needed. The examination should include the use of the standard questionnaire relating to the characteristic symptoms of byssinosis as well as the more common symptoms of chronic non-specific chest disease, and, as an essential, a simple test of ventilatory capacity of the lungs such as the $FEV_{1\cdot 0}$ and the Forced Vital Capacity (FVC). The $FEV_{1\cdot 0}$/FVC ratio falls in obstructive lung disease and may be a more useful measure of expiratory resistance than the FEV alone and has the advantage of being independent of weight (Valić *et al.*, 1968). The change of ventilatory capacity during a work shift by recording the $FEV_{1 \cdot 0}$ before and after exposure to dust will detect workers who are particularly susceptible to the dust. This test should preferably be done on the first day back at work.

Periodic examinations should be at intervals of not more than 3 years. Where dust concentrations exceed 1 mg/M^3 less fly the interval should be one year. Workers showing a marked fall in ventilatory capacity either during the shift or between one examination and another, or having severe symptoms of byssinosis should be moved to less dusty jobs unless immediate steps can be taken to control the dust in the workplace. Individual protection in the form of face masks or fresh air hoods may be necessary in maintenance work, where high exposure to high dust concentrations is often inevitable.

The complete eradication of byssinosis by the removal of toxic dust from the workrooms is not yet in sight. But a combination of environmental control and medical surveillance could in the future prevent most, if not all, workers at risk being severely disabled.

References

Barbero, A. and Flores, R. (1944), "Enfermedad del canamo." *Rev. Clin. Esp.*, **13**, 395.

Bouhuys, A., Barbero, A., Lindell, S. E., Roach, S. A. and Schilling, R. S. F. (1967), "Byssinosis in Hemp Workers." *Arch. Envir. Hlth.*, **14**, 533.

Bouhuys, A., Barbero, A., Schilling, R. S. F. and van de Woestigne, K. P. (1969), "Cigarette Smoking, Occupational Dust Exposure and Ventilatory Capacity." *Amer. J. Med.*, **46**, 526.

Bouhuys, A., Gilson, J. G. and Schilling, R. S. F. (1970), "Byssinosis in the Textile Industry." *Arch. Envir. Hlth.*, **21**, 475.

Bouhuys, A., Heaphy, L. J., Schilling, R. S. F. and Wellborn, J. W. (1967), "Byssinosis in the United States." *New. Eng. J. Med.*, **277**, 170.

Bouhuys, A. (1966), "Byssinosis in Textile Workers." *Trans. N.Y. Acad. Sci.*, **28**, p. 480.

British Medical Journal (1962), "World Wide Byssinosis." **2**, 781.

British Occupational Hygiene Society (1972), "Hygiene Standards for Cotton Dust" (to be published).

Carey, G. C. R., Elwood, P. C., McAuley, I. R., Merrett, J. D. and Pemberton, J. (1965), *Byssinosis in Flax and Hemp Workers.* Ministry of Pensions and National Insurance. H.M.S.O. (Cmnd. 2730).

Cotes, J. E. (1968), "Lung Function." Blackwell, Oxford.

El Batawi and Hussein, M. (1964), "Endemic Byssinosis in an Egyptian Village." *Brit. J. Indust. Med.*, **21**, 231.

El Batawi, M., Schilling, R. S. F., Valić, F. and Walford, J. (1964), "Byssinosis in the Egyptian Cotton Industry." *Brit. J. Indust. Med.*, **21**, 13.

Gilson, J. (1968), Personal Communication at International Conference on Byssinosis, Alicante.

Hitchcock, M., Piscitelli, D. M. and Bouhuys, A. (1971). "Hislamine release from human lung by 48/80 and methyl piperonylate". *Proc. Int. Cong. Phys. Sciences.* Munich p. 251.

Lammers, B., Schilling, R. S. F. and Walford, J. (1964), "A Study of Byssinosis in English and Dutch Cotton Workers." *Brit. J. Indust. Med.*, **21,** 124.

Massoud, A. and Taylor, G. (1964), "Byssinosis: Antibody to cotton antigens in Normal Subjects and in Cotton Card Room Workers." *Lancet*, **2,** 607.

McKerrow, C., Gilson, J., Schilling, R. S. F. and Skidmore, J. W. (1965), "Respiratory Function and Symptoms in Rope Workers." *Brit. J. Indust. Med.*, **22,** 204.

McKerrow, C., McDermott, M., Gilson, J. and Schilling, R. S. F. (1958), "Respiratory Function During the Day in Cotton Workers: A Study in Byssinosis. *Brit. J. Indust. Med.*, **15,** 75.

McKerrow, C., Roach, S. A., Gilson, J. C. and Schilling, R. S. F. (1962), "The Size of Cotton Dust Particles causing Byssinosis." *Brit. J. Indust. Med.*, **19,** 1.

Mekky, S., Roach, S. A. and Schilling, R. S. F. (1967), "Byssinosis amongst Winders in the Cotton Industry." *Brit. J. Indust. Med.*, **24,** 132.

Molyneux, M. K. B. and Tombleson, J. B. L. (1970), "An Epidemiological Study of Respiratory Symptoms in Lancashire Mills, 1963–66." *Brit. J. Indust. Med.*, **27,** 225.

Munt, D. F., Gauvain, S., Walford, J. and Schilling, R. S. F. (1965), "Study of Respiratory Symptoms and Ventilatory Capacities among Rope Workers." *Brit. J. Indust. Med.*, **22,** 196.

Nicholls, P. J., Nicholls, G. R. and Bouhuys, A. (1966), *Histamine Release by Compound* 48/80 *and Textile Dusts from Lung Tissue in Vitro. Inhaled Particles and Vapours* II, p. 69. Ed. C. N. Davies. London: Pergamon Press.

Patissier, P. (1822), *Traite des Maladies des Artisans.* Paris: J. B. Balliere, 1940.

Ramazzini, B. (1713), *Diseases of Workers.* Latin Text of 1713, revised with translation and notes by W. C. Wright. Chicago University Press, 1940.

Roach, S. A. and Schilling, R. S. F. (1960), "A Clinical and Environmental Study of Byssinosis in the Lancashire Cotton Industry." *Brit. J. Indust. Med.*, **17,** 1.

Schilling, R. S. F. (1962), "Case Study No. 2: Field Studies of Byssinosis." *J. Occ. Med.*, **4,** 627.

Schilling, R. S. F. (1964), "Epidemiological Studies of Chronic Respiratory Disease among Cotton Operatives." *Yale J. Biol. Med.*, **37,** 1.

Schilling, R. S. F. (1956), "Byssinosis in Cotton and other Textile Workers." *Lancet*, **2,** 261 and 319.

Schilling, R. S. F., Vigliani, E. C., Lammers, B., Valić, F. and Gilson, J. C. (1963), *Proceedings of the XIV International Congress on Occupational Health, Madrid.* Reprinted from the *Excerpta Medica International Congress on Occ. Health No.* 62.

Smith, G. F., Coles, G. V., Schilling, R. S. F. and Walford, J. (1969), "A study of Rope Workers Exposed to Hemp Flax." *Brit. J. Indust. Med.*, **26,** 109.

Taylor, G., Massoud, A. and Lucas, F. (1971), "Studies on the Aetiology of Byssinosis." *Brit. J. Indust. Med.*, **28,** 143.

Tiller, J. R. and Schilling, R. S. F. (1958), "Respiratory Function During the Day in Rayon Workers: A study in Byssinosis." *Trans. Assoc. Indust. Med. Officers*, **7,** 161.

Valić, F., Žuškin, E., Walford, J., Keršić, W. and Pauković, R. (1968), "Byssinosis, Chronic Bronchitis and Ventilatory Capacity among Rope Workers." *Brit. J. Indust. Med.*, **25,** 196.

Walford, J., Lammers, B. and Schilling, R. S. F. (with D. Van Hoven van Genderen and Y. G. van der Veen). (1966), "Diurnal Variation in Ventilatory Capacity." *Brit. J. Indust. Med.*, **23,** 142.

Žuškin, E., Wolfson, R., Harpel, G., Welborn, J. W. and Bouhuys, A. (1969), "Byssinosis in Carding and Spinning Workers." *Arch. Envir. Hlth.*, **19,** 166.

Chapter 6

Asbestos

P. C. Elmes

"IV. Inventum iam est etiam quod ignibus non absumeretur. vivum id vocant, ardentesque in focis conviviorum ex eo vidimus mappas sordibus exustio splendescentes igni magis quam possent aquis. regum inde funebres tunicae corporis favillam ab reliquo separant cinere. nascitur in desertis adustisque Indiae locis, ubi non cadunt imbres, inter dires serpentes, adsuescitque vivere ardendo, rarum in ventu, difficile textu propter brevitatem; rufus de cetero colos splendescit igni. cum inventum est aequat pretia excellentium margaritarum vocatur autem a Graecis *σβεστινου* ex argumento naturae suae."

Pliny

"IV. Also a linen has now been invented that is incombustible. It is called 'live' linen, and I have seen napkins made of it glowing on the hearth at banquets and burnt more brilliantly clean by the fire than they could be by being washed in water. This linen is used for making shrouds for royalty which keep the ashes of the corpse separate from the rest of the pyre. The plant grows in the deserts and sun-scorched regions of India where no rain falls, the haunts of deadly snakes, and it is habituated to living in burning heat; it is rarely found, and is difficult to weave into cloth because of its shortness; its colour is normally red but turns white by the action of fire. When any of it is found, it rivals the prices of exceptionally fine pearls. The Greek name for it is asbestinon, derived from its peculiar property."

Although the word asbestos means unquenchable in classical Greek it is obvious from Pliny's use of it that it was already used to describe non inflammable cloth and the raw material from which this was made. Agricola (1546) points out that in classical Greek and Roman times material which seems to have been asbestos was described by a number of names such as "amiantus" because it is not destroyed by fire, "bostrychites" because it is braided like hair and "carystium" because one of the mines was near Carystos in Euboea. It is evident that asbestos, as we understand it now, was used in ancient times and that by Agricola's day it was used in lamp wicks and fire resistant cloth in much the same way as it is sometimes used today. The word asbestos is now used as a descriptive term for any fibrous silicate mineral used commercially because of its resistance to heat and chemicals.

During the second half of the industrial revolution the demand for more efficient power units led to the development of larger furnaces and boilers and high pressure steam supplying double or triple expansion engines. The presence of high temperature steam pipes in the confines of locomotives and steam boats became recognized as a hazard which ordinary cloth, cork or wood insulation did not prevent. The sudden demand for safer insulation material was more than the old asbestos

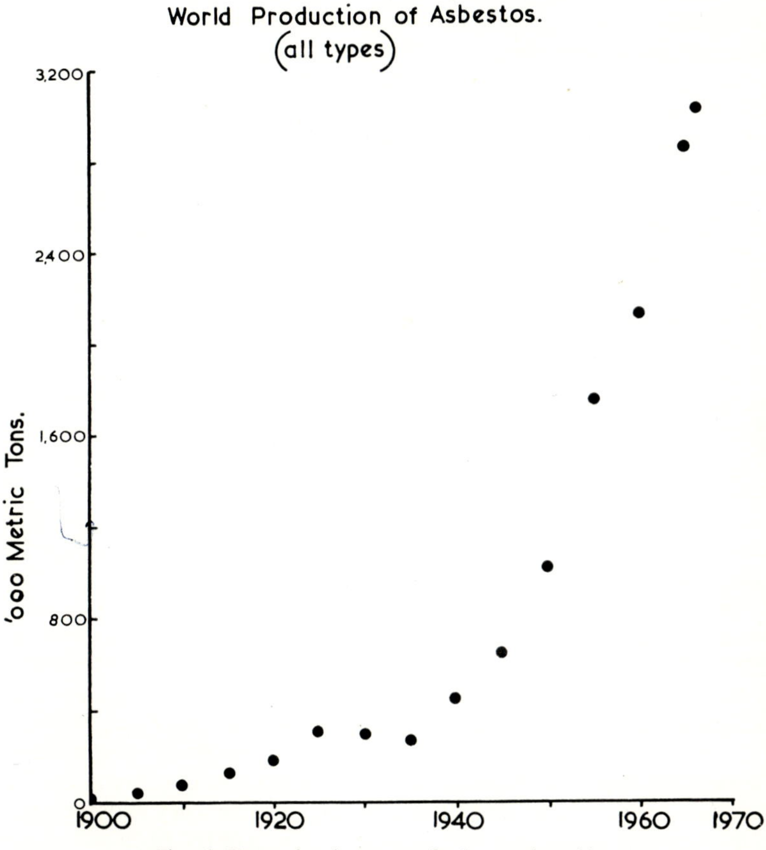

FIG. 1. Expansion in usage of asbestos (graph). Material supplied by Holmes (1969) from various sources.

mines in Finland, Germany and Northern Italy could meet. It was fortuitous that large and relatively easily mined deposits were found in South Africa and Canada in the last half of the 19th century. Cheap asbestos became available and output was expanded rapidly to meet demand (see Fig. 1). At first asbestos was only used for insulation, either as stuffed cloth quilts or as a plaster made up with magnesia. But such a strong, cheap and relatively inert fibrous material soon found other uses. Since the recognition of the danger to health in 1930, changing technology in industry has caused a great increase in the use of asbestos apparently unhampered, until recently, by health considerations.

The Minerals

The collective term asbestos is used for a group of silicate minerals which have re-crystallized into long fibres. Chrysotile was formed in the cracks of the hard rock serpentine. The other commercial asbestos fibres are amphiboles and formed in sedimentary ironstones, probably in the floor of early lakes or seas. They were all formed by re-crystallization of the constituents dissolved from the parent rock by water at a high temperature and pressure (Fig. 2). They are estimated to have formed about 2,000 million years ago and were thought to have preceded the appearance of living organisms on earth. However, recent evidence (Harington, 1962) derived from the study of organic oils and waxes which are associated with asbestos ore has been taken to suggest pre-existing living matter. There are two molecular lattices concerned and in both of them sheets of hexagonally packed silica units are sandwiched between sheets of cation oxide.

Chrysotile has the more complex lattice structure. The silica sheets are linked to sheets of magnesium hydroxide (brucite) by the substitution of oxygen atoms projecting from the silica for the hydroxyl groups of the brucite. Because the mesh of the silica lattice is slightly smaller than that of the brucite, the pairs of sheets are curved with the silica on the inside, and in well formed fibres the sheets are rolled up like a scroll of parchment (Fig. 3). Thus a typical chrysotile fibre is 500 Å in diameter, with a 60 Å hole down the middle made up ten layers of paired sheets. As the disparity between the lattices of the two sheets is not completely satisfied by curvature in a single plane, there is usually some curvature in the other plane leading to the spiral or wavy appearance of the fibres. In the rock and as used commercially the spaces between the fibres are filled with less well oriented silica and brucite units. There is also a quantity of oxides of iron and calcium and traces of other metals. These other ions are characteristic of a given ore but there is marked variation from mine to mine. It is not clear whether they may form part of the lattice structure and help to improve the fit of the silica and brucite sheets or whether they simply get caught up in the spaces between and down the centre of the scrolls (Speil and Leineweber, 1968).

Crocidolite (riebeckite), amosite (cummingtonite) and anthophyllite are the other commercially important asbestos minerals. They are all amphiboles and share a common lattice structure. The pairs of silica sheets are sandwiched between flat plates of cation oxide. There seems no limit to the number of plates which build up in this way or to their width. But this group of amphiboles cleave easily both by separation of the sheets and along their length. This basic structure explains the fact that amphibole asbestos fibres tend to be straight but coarser (800 to

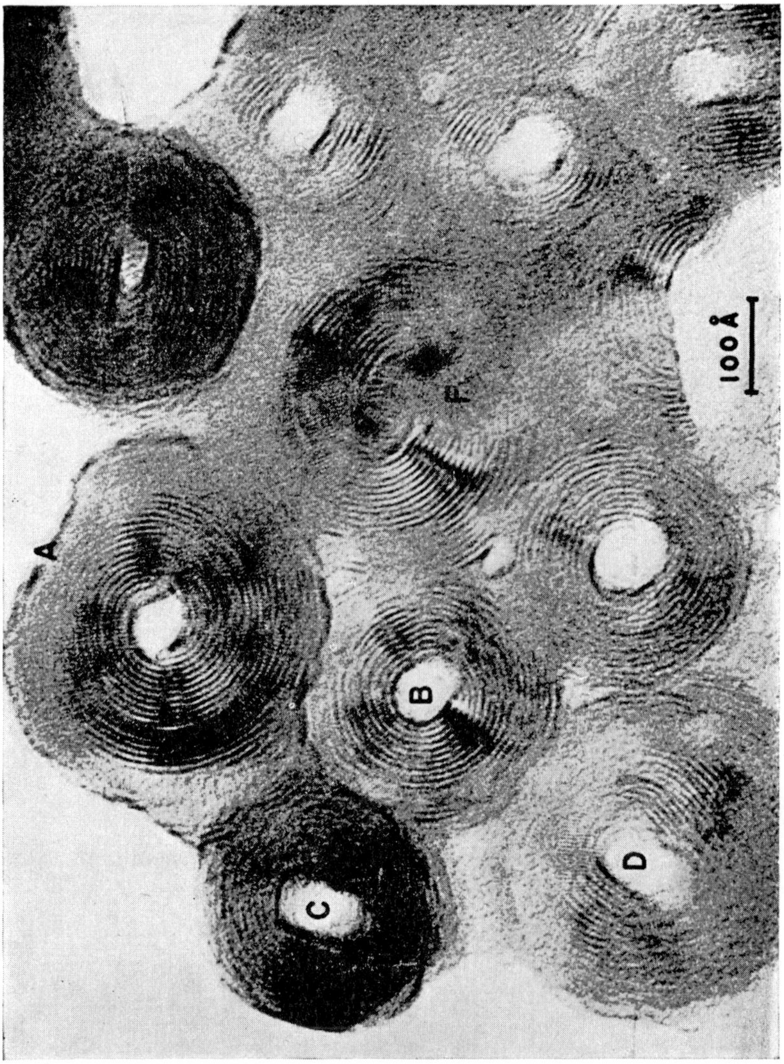

FIG. 3. Scroll structure of chrysotile asbestos. Electromicrograph of cross section (Yada, 1967).
(Reprinted from *Acta Crystallographica.* Vol. 23, p. 704–707. Plate 15 (Fig. 7).)

1,000 Å in diameter) and more variable in cross section than the curved scrolls of chrysotile. The amphiboles differ in the cation constituents of the cation layer of the crystals. Although (see Table 1) fixed formulae are given there is in fact some variation in the content of ferric, ferrous,

Table 1
Kinds of asbestos in commercial use

Name	*Formula and Geological Name*	*Percentage of world production**
Chrysotile	$Mg_3(Si_2O_5)(OH)_4$ Chrysotile	93
Crocidolite "Blue"	$Na_2Fe_3{}^{++}Fe_2{}^{+++}(Si_8O_{22})(OH,F)_2$ Riebeckite	3·5
Amosite	$(Mg, Fe^{++})_7(Si_8O_{22})(OH)_2$ Cummingtonite	2·4
Anthophyllite	$(Mg, Fe^{++})_7(Si_8O_{22})(OH,F)_2$ Anthophyllite (always mixed with Gedrite)	1·1†

* Estimated Total Production (1962) 3·2 million tons
† Including actinolite and tremolite

sodium and magnesium ions between samples of the individual ores. There are also traces of potassium, manganese and other metals as well as oils and waxes which may be present as inclusions from the mother liquor.

Related minerals such as the talcs often cleave in a fibrous manner and give rise to dust, which is in effect asbestos, when they are handled mechanically.

These minerals are associated with solid rocks which may have an identical chemical and X-ray crystallographic structure, but, because of differences in temperature and pressure, did not recrystallize into long fibrous forms.

Epidemiological studies (see below) have suggested important differences between the hazards produced by the various commercial forms of asbestos. They have certain individual characteristics (see Table 2) which makes it relatively easy to distinguish them in the pure

Table 2
Microscopic characteristics of fibres

Name	*Colour*	*Sign of birefringence*	*Extinction angle*	*Mean diameter*
Chrysotile	White to grey green	+ve	90°	150–400 Å
Crocidolite	Blue	−ve	90 ∓ 3°	800–1000 Å
Amosite	White to brown	+ve	90 ± 15°	1000 Å
Anthophyllite	Green to brown	+ve	90°	1000 Å

state. But no practical method has been devised for distinguishing between these fibres as they appear in the dust of a factory or in the lung of a patient. The features in polarized light microscopy (the negative sign of birefringence of the crocidolite and inclined extinction angle of the amosite) are impossible to identify when fragments 2–3 μ

long and embedded in organic material are being examined in random orientation. The only sure identification is the recognition of the scroll structure of the chrysotile. This requires electron microscopy. As yet X-ray diffraction and electron probes have not been used in a way suitable for quantitative analysis of large numbers of specimens of mixed dusts.

Uses

All forms of asbestos are relatively tough, inert and resistant to both heat and chemicals. The differences noted in Table 3 are only relative

Table 3

Physical and chemical characteristics of fibres

Name	*Water of crystallization*	*Tensile strength (lbs/sq. in.)*	*Heat resistance*	*Acid resistance*
Chrysotile	14%	350,000	Good	Relatively soluble
Crocidolite	2%	500,000	Relatively poor	Very good
Amosite	2%	175,000	Good	Good
Anthophyllite	2%	100,000	Very good	Good

(Gaze, 1965.)

and govern the commercial choice for extreme conditions. In practice it is the availability, cost and ease of handling that governs the commercial use of these compounds for most purposes. The large easily-worked deposits of chrysotile in Eastern Canada and in Russia are the most convenient source of asbestos for North America and the Iron Curtain countries respectively. It is because of this geographical and economic linkage that chrysotile production exceeds that of the other fibres by such a wide margin.

Chrysotile is rather better for textile manufacture because it can yield fibres up to 3 in. long and can be spun easily without breaking. The shorter fibre chrysotile can be used as a strengthener in cement products and as a filler in plastics, particularly floor tiles. Amosite is too brittle to weave but is much used in plaster insulation. Crocidolite is used preferentially when its resistance to acid is valuable.

Asbestos cement products such as corrugated roofing, drain pipe, wall and ceiling boards and mixes for cement floors, cladding of steel building framework, etc., consume in about two-thirds of the world output of all types of asbestos. Many insurance companies and fire authorities stipulate a content of asbestos in building materials to delay the heat failure of the steel framework and the spread of fire through modern buildings. Related to this is the use of asbestos as a filler and strengthener in caulking mastics and paints. Filling for floor tiles and other plastics and special paper consumes the second largest quantity of asbestos and the manufacture of brake linings and pads and gaskets for cars, etc., is the next. Although asbestos cloth quilts filled with teased asbestos fibre are not often used to insulate boilers now, asbestos textiles still account for about one-fiftieth of the world consumption. Glass fibre, both woven and felted is replacing asbestos for many purposes where the temperature range is not excessive. Asbestos is still used in lamp wicks but not for table napkins or shrouds.

Changing technology is constantly finding new uses for this strong, cheap, relatively inert fibrous mineral.

Sources of Exposure

Asbestos is only a source of danger if it penetrates the tissues of the body, and it is when suspended in the air as a respirable dust that this is most likely to occur.

Natural Weathering

In areas where asbestos containing rocks are naturally exposed and fragmented the soil may contain fibres of respirable size. In Bulgaria, where tobacco is grown in such mountainous areas, the lungs of agricultural workers have shown minor evidence of asbestos exposure (Zolov, Burilkov and Babadjov, 1968; Burilkov and Michailova, 1970). Unless a similar process contributes to the incidence of mesothelioma in South Africa there is no proof that natural weathering is a serious source of exposure.

Mining and Milling

The ease of extraction of asbestos from the ground depends on the hardness of the parent rock. Much of the amphibole asbestos is mined by open cast or quarrying methods which cause a great deal of contamination of the surrounding countryside. The use of rock residues still containing some asbestos as aggregate for building roads and railways makes this problem worse. Studies around the crocidolite mines in South Africa (Wagner, Sleggs and Marchand, 1960) and the anthophyllite mines in Finland (Kiviluoto, 1965) show that environmental exposure can be very extensive.

The dust produced by this type of mining and quarrying is rapidly dispersed by the wind so that the working men may have little more exposure than the surrounding population. But in the deeper mines in harder rock needed to gain chrysotile the exposure to the miner is correspondingly greater and that of the rest of the population less. In most mining areas the crude rock is milled and the asbestos separated and partially teased out in open mills at or close to the mine. Little effort has been made to suppress dust in these processes up until recently. Workmen and neighbourhood populations are exposed. The hand separation of asbestos from its parent rock (cobbing) by cheap labour and the use of tips as playgrounds for children has added to the population at risk, especially in the South African mining areas.

It was the practice to transport asbestos from the mines to the primary users in Hessian bags which gave off a cloud of asbestos dust whenever they were handled. As a result a whole chain of transport workers, dockers and labourers have been exposed intermittently and there is evidence that these men, and the women employed repairing these sacks, have had clinically significant exposure (Owen, 1965). This risk can be eliminated by the use of impervious paper or plastic sealed bags which are not re-used. The same applies to the transport of waste asbestos material and lagging which has stripped off. Tips for such waste can be a source of wind-blown dust if not properly sited and covered.

Manufacturing

Asbestos factories can be classified into two main groups—those producing asbestos cement materials such as corrugated sheeting, pipes and other building materials, and those producing asbestos textile materials. These primary industries produce few ordinary consumer goods; their products are used in secondary industrial processes and in building. In this way two groups of industrial workers may become exposed to asbestos, those making the cement products or textiles and those using the products in building or in the manufacture of cars, lamps, stoves, etc. In an intermediate position are the store-keepers and warehousemen who handle the products of primary industry and groups of workers such as pipe laggers who use materials only partially processed by the primary industry for insulation work.

In secondary industry there are small groups of men who saw or machine an asbestos component all day so that they are as much at risk as the men in the primary industry. But on the whole the risk of exposure is greatest in the primary industry, less in the intermediate group and least in the user or secondary industry.

Use of Completed Products

Much has been written in the lay press about the dangers created by certain asbestos containing products in the environment of the community, the wear of motor car brake linings, the weathering of asbestos roofing, the flaking off of asbestos from ceiling tiles and, more particularly, from the asbestos coating used on the insides of roofs and air ducts. This last material is sprayed on with water, a process known as limpet spraying, and creates a loosely-bound thick layer containing 80–90% asbestos fibre, which protects against the condensation of moisture as well as against fire.

It is highly probable that these and many other asbestos-containing objects do contribute to a certain level of general atmosphere pollution and that this may be rather higher in certain buildings where unsealed asbestos has been used in the air conditioning and ventilating systems. What is not yet known is whether the levels of contamination are of clinical significance.

What may be much more important is the intermittent exposure encountered by the maintenance engineer, the electrician, painters and joiners who have to work in asbestos-lined duct spaces or drill holes in asbestos building materials during their work. The same applies to the home handyman and tradesman who re-wires his house, puts in central heating and does other jobs and may use sheet material containing asbestos without being aware of the risk involved.

Destruction and Demolition

In the repair and maintenance of boilers and steam pipes in ships, it has always been the job of the insulation worker to strip off old insulation and then re-apply new when the repair job has been completed. The breaking off of old dry "boiler compound" and similar insulation is a very dusty procedure contributing to the hazard to which insulation workers are exposed. But particularly in the demolition of factories and offices, there is no such job specialization and demolition workers may get heavy temporary exposure and produce neighbourhood contamination without being aware that they are creating a hazard.

Biological Effects of Asbestos

Mode of Entry. This is almost entirely by inhalation, but dust can also get in on food and through cuts and abrasions. In the past it has been deliberately inserted into the body during surgical procedures. Peritoneal mesotheliomas and the increased incidence of gastrointestinal cancer in groups exposed to asbestos (see below) may be due to food contamination, but they could also arise from the migration of fibres from the lungs or from swallowed sputum. Men who handle asbestos continually get "asbestos warts", benign hyperkeratotic lesions where asbestos has rubbed into a cut. These subside when the foreign body is removed and there is no evidence as to whether asbestos can migrate to other sites as a result of this type of lesion. Talc used on surgeons' gloves is now known to be contaminated with "asbestos" fibres although the French claim that their product is free from fibrous material (Avril, 1968). Talc granulomas are well known and have always been attributed to the talc rather than to the contaminating asbestos. But asbestos was deliberately inserted by certain surgeons into the pericardium in the surgical treatment of angina and talc has been used in a similar way in the treatment of recurrent pneumothorax. The long-term follow-up of these cases would be very interesting in the light of present knowledge.

Particle Size and Retention in the Lung

Asbestos dust consists of bundles of fibres varying in length and in the number of constituent fibres. Therefore there is a great variation in both the size and thickness of the particles depending on the amount of teasing that has already occurred and the impact speeds creating the dust. When crude ore and asbestos cement materials are being handled there is contamination with other dusts which may also be pathogenic.

Elongated particles sediment more slowly in air than non fibrous particles because the sedimentation of dust depends on the minimal cross sectional area rather than length or weight. Therefore bundles of asbestos fibres form a stable, respirable dust up to fibre lengths of 2–300 μ. There is no clear cut lower end to the range of particle sizes which can be retained in the lung. It has been shown experimentally (Timbrell and Skidmore, 1968) that when mixed asbestos clouds are inhaled by animals a larger proportion of the fibres over 20 μ in length are retained. But in asbestos clouds there is always a far greater number of fibres of under 20 μ in length and even under 5 μ. In these experiments, in spite of the preferential absorption of long fibres, the bulk of the fibres retained were short. Examination of experimental material with the electron microscope reveals large quantities of very small fragments retained in the lung.

Chrysotile fibre bundles are curved and, although this does not affect the sedimentation in air to an appreciable extent, it may affect retention in the lung. A curved fibre will not get so far down the bronchial tree before it is caught on the bronchial wall and removed by ciliary action. Therefore fewer large chrysotile fibres will be retained. This may be part of the explanation for the difference in the epidemiological findings between chrysotile and other asbestos dusts.

Up to the present time human data relating morbidity to dust exposure has not been analysed for fibre size. Even current dust measurements only record fibres between 5 and 100 microns in length so that it will be a long time before such information will be available (Roach, 1968). Analysis of fibre length in human lung is not of great help because there is evidence that over the years asbestos fragments into shorter and shorter particles in the lung (Knox and Beattie, 1954).

The Effect of Asbestos Dust on the Lungs

Human material tends to reveal only the end result of asbestos exposure so that knowledge of the pathogenesis of the lung lesions depends on animal studies. In order to produce changes within the life span of laboratory animals it has been the practice to use very intense exposure; this difference and the species differences make the application of experimental findings to human experience difficult. But on the whole the end result of dust exposure of rats, guinea pigs (Holt, Mills and

Young, 1964–5) and dogs (McIver, 1968) resembles the asbestosis produced by heavy exposure in man.

The larger fibres retained in the lung lodge in the terminal bronchiole and penetrate the tissues at this point. There is a macrophage response as well as haemorrhage with lysis of the red cells in the tissues. These longer fibres do not migrate towards the hilum in lymphatics but tend

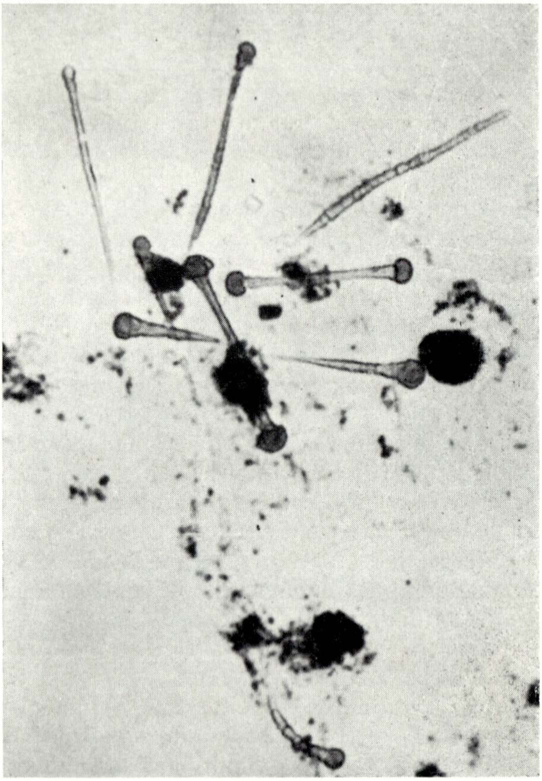

FIG. 4.

(a) Asbestos bodies

to migrate towards the subpleural tissue and accumulate there. Because of the length of the fibres, individual macrophages can only engulf a small part of the length of any one bundle of fibres which may be attacked by several macrophages at once. Within a few days (Botham and Holt, 1968a) a protein iron complex is laid down around some of the fibres by the macrophages to form asbestos bodies. This coating is similar to ferritin (Davis, 1964); it resembles clear amber and stains positively for iron. It has a characteristic appearance (Figs. 4 and 5) which identifies the asbestos body in the bulk of clinical material.

Similar bodies can form around other foreign particles in the lung but usually the core is opaque, black and irregular. However, Botham and Holt (1968b) have shown recently that glass fibres of the right order of thickness will produce bodies indistinguishable from asbestos bodies. The experimental studies have not solved two problems associated with the inhalation of relatively long asbestos bodies. Firstly not all

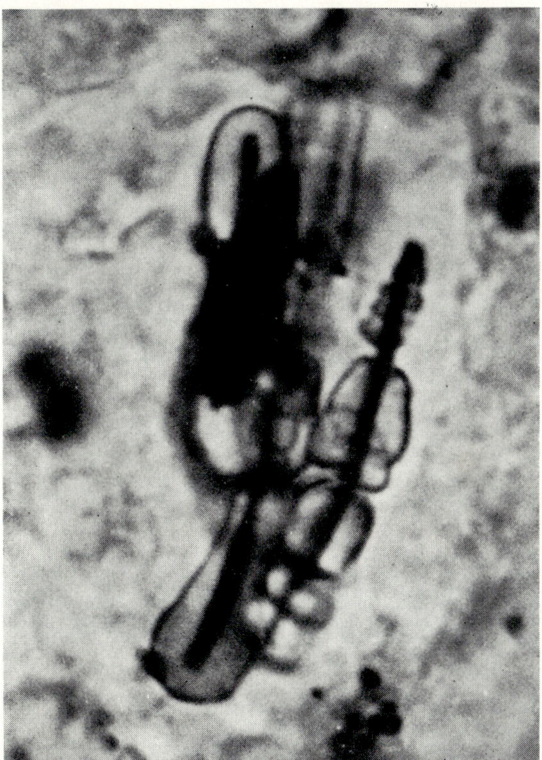

FIG. 4.
(b) Ferruginous bodies formed from other material

fibres become coated. The proportion coated varies from species to species and also depends on the mode of entry. Guinea-pigs form bodies readily around inhaled fibres but rats form very few unless the asbestos is inserted into the tissues or a serous cavity. In human material there are always more uncoated fibres than bodies. Secondly, there is the problem of biological activity. Freshly inserted or inhaled material provokes the haemorrhage and macrophage reaction followed by fibrosis of the interstitial tissue of the lung. But even in the relatively short period of the animal studies this evidence of activity ceases and other

(a)

(b)

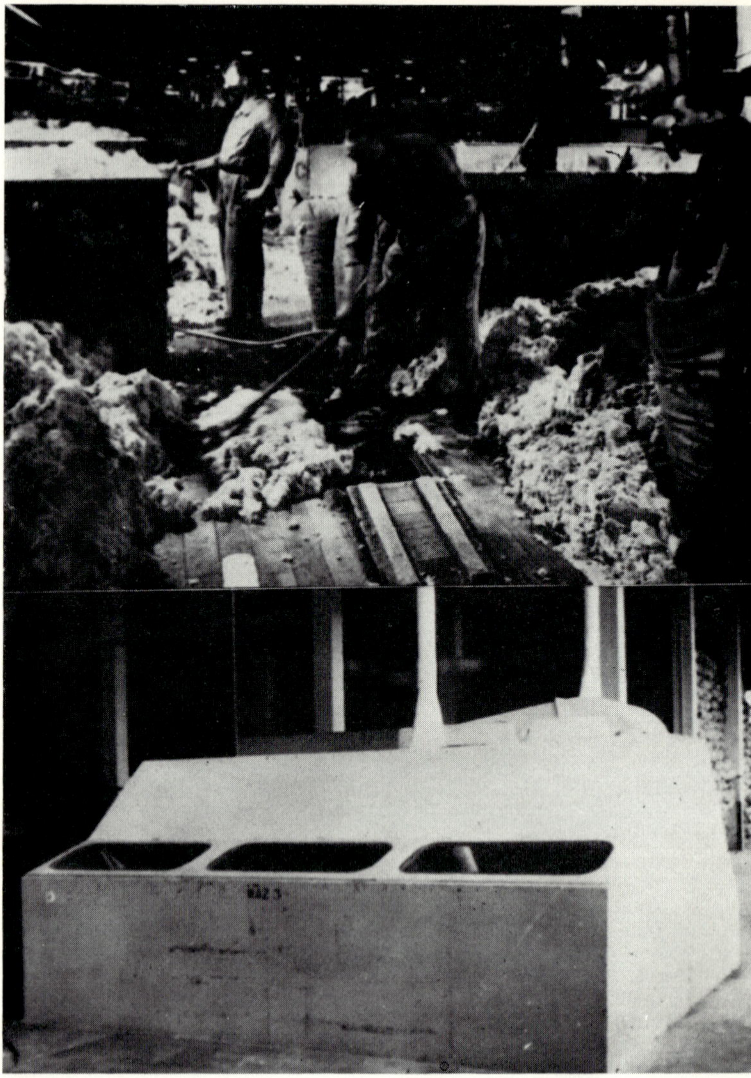

FIG. 5.

(a) Mixing asbestos as it was done before 1931 (except masks were not worn)

(b) Enclosed mixing machine

uncoated and coated fibres seem to remain as inert foreign bodies. Beattie and Knox (1961) have commented on this in relation to human material and suggest that it is only when asbestos fibres are first inhaled, and later when both the uncoated fibres and asbestos bodies break up after many years that they are biologically active.

Short fibres landing in the airways are probably removed in the bronchial mucus and either swallowed or expectorated. If they land in the alveolus they are taken up by alveolar macrophages and even true alveolar epithelial cells (Suzuki, Chung and Smith, 1968). The fibres are taken into the macrophages in phagosomes but these may rupture leaving the fibre free in the cytoplasm. The macrophages coalesce to form giant cells (Davis, 1968) which become the centre of a granulomatous reaction. In the guinea-pig exposed intensively to small fibres this leads to carnification and progressive fibrosis of the alveolar part of the lung (Holt *et al.*, 1965). In the hamster there is a reversion of the alveolar epithelium toward the cuboidal pattern found in the foetus (Suzuki *et al.*, 1968). This type of transformation is seen in human material where there is fibrosis of the alveolar wall.

Klosterkötter (1968) has pointed out the difficulty of interpreting the experimental findings with short fibres in terms of human disease because of the different sizes of fibre and sizes of animal used by different workers. However, all workers agree that polyvinyl pyridin-n-oxide does not prevent the fibrosis produced by asbestos in the way it prevents experimental silicosis.

Ultimate fate of Fibres

Once the initial reaction has subsided the fibres and asbestos bodies appear to behave like inert foreign bodies. Asbestos bodies have been found in such widely distributed human tissues as the brain and the kidney. But whether they move as formed bodies or as fibres which become bodies when they reach that final destination is not known. Recent experimental studies by Holmes and Morgan (1968) using irradiated material indicate that the fibres migrate about the body while at the same time they fragment and dissolve so that their break-down products are excreted. Uncoated fibres are difficult to detect in the tissues especially if they are small and asbestos bodies are not present to draw attention to them. So that, although this dissemination may occur in humans with inhalation exposure, the extent to which it occurs and its contribution to the effects of exposure is not known. Differences between the clinical effects of different kinds of asbestos may be due to differences in the proportion of fibres forming asbestos bodies and the rate of migration and disintegration of the fibres. Only fragmentary evidence is available as yet.

Human Experience

(i) **Early conditions.** Early industrialists had no inkling of the dangers of exposing their employees to this dust. The chemical inertness and physical indestructibility which made asbestos so useful suggested that the material would be safe and would not carry the hazards already described for flax and cotton because of the virtual absence of organic material. Asbestos was teased out, bagged, spun, woven, machined and cut in open crude machines in poorly ventilated factories. Not only those employed on the dusty job but everyone else in the factory was exposed. In the early days the workers thought nothing of putting girls into the hemp sacks full of asbestos dust. Even now it is difficult to stop shipyard workers from playing football with disintegrating lagging material on decks of unventilated ships. This sort of lunch-hour horseplay indicates the attitude of many towards the hazard of inhaling asbestos dust.

Realization of the hazard has come in two stages, first the lung fibrosis and second the development of cancer. The first stage began in 1900 when a man of 33 who had spent 14 years carding asbestos, died of a pulmonary fibrosis. Dr. Montague Murray (1907) gave evidence before a Departmental Committee to the effect that this pulmonary fibrosis was due to exposure to asbestos. He also related that 10 other men who were already doing the same work when the patient started had all died before the patient. A proper epidemiological study was *not* carried out and after asking the Trades Union Congress for their opinion the Committee reported that there was insufficient evidence to include asbestos in the list of hazardous industrial materials. However, the Home Office surveyed the industry in 1910 and arranged for Professor Beattie in Sheffield to carry out some studies with guinea-pigs. Although Professor Beattie showed that the dust caused pulmonary fibrosis experimentally the Home Office failed to find evidence of a serious hazard in the industry (Merewether and Price, 1930).

The high incidence of pulmonary tuberculosis particularly among young women in the general population, no doubt accounts for the fact that the high mortality amongst young workers first employed in asbestos factories during the first war was not attributed to this dust exposure. Cases were described in this era and in retrospect it is hard to realize why it was not until Seiler's (1928) well documented case that a fuller investigation of the industry was carried out.

(ii) **Merewether's Investigation.** Dr. Merewether, on behalf of the Factory Department, concentrated on the asbestos textile industry. Here the dust was mainly asbestos whereas in the asbestos cement industry it would have been difficult to differentiate the contribution of the other dusts.

In the whole sample of 363 workers employed in 1930, 26% had radiological fibrosis. But among those exposed for over 20 years, 80% had fibrosis while those exposed less than 5 years had none. In the dustiest occupations symptoms developed in 7–9 years and death could occur after only 12 years.

The "Merewether" report (Merewether and Price, 1930) led to the recognition of pulmonary fibrosis (asbestosis) due to asbestos as an industrial hazard and certain regulations concerning dust control and the protection and supervision of workers were issued. Because the survey concerned asbestos textile workers the regulations were only applied to textile factories and to similar processes in the cement factories. For lack of evidence the regulations were not applied to the rest of the asbestos cement industry or to user industries. Insulation workers were not kept under statutory medical supervision. Public awareness of the hazard did lead to some doubts as to the adequacy of the regulations, letters appeared in the medical journals and questions were asked in Parliament as to the safety both to the workers themselves and to members of the public of such processes as the limpet spraying of the inner surface of London Tube tunnels. These questions had as little effect in protecting insulation workers as the efforts made after Montague Murray's case had in protecting factory workers in 1906.

(iii) **Asbestosis.** *The pathology*. The prescription of asbestosis as an industrial disease had as one of its effects the follow-up of all workers in certain prescribed occupations until their death. After death the coroner had to be notified and in a high proportion of cases an autopsy was carried out. This meant that the cause of death and the pattern of pathological change in this group became accurately established. At

Table 4

Changes in postmortem findings in workers in an asbestos factory
(After Smither, 1965.)

	1931–49	1957–64
Number of deaths	115	71
Age	40·8	56
Tuberculosis	36	4*
Carcinoma of the lung	17	26
Primary pleural and peritoneal malignancy	1	15
Other abdominal malignancy	7	7

* All inactive.

first the high incidence of tuberculosis (see Table 4) made the interpretation of the findings difficult, but as the frequency of tuberculosis declined it became easier to define the effects of asbestos on the lungs of these factory workers. As far as is known the description which follows is true for all forms of asbestos exposure sufficiently heavy to cause radiological fibrosis before the end of the working life. The picture in the asbestos cement and some of the other industries may be complicated by the presence of other dusts. Little is known about the comparative pathology of the various industrial and mining communities. Speculation has arisen recently about the interaction between inhaled dusts and other diseases (rheumatoid arthritis) and other inhaled material. Evidence that a similar relationship exists between the response to asbestos and the presence of auto-antibodies is now accumulating (Turner-Warwick, 1970).

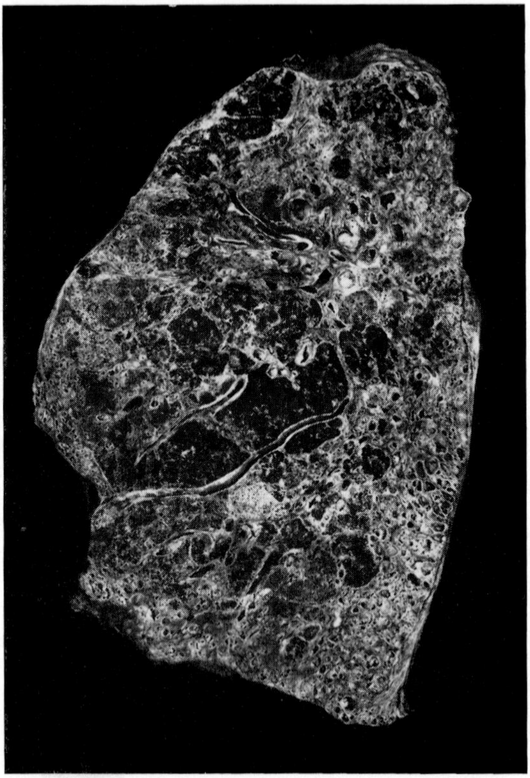

FIG. 6. Severe asbestosis showing areas of honeycomb change in a woman employed filling asbestos quilts for 12 years.

The Lung

The advanced case shows a diffuse fibrosis of lung and pleura making the lungs smaller and stiffer than normal. The shrinkage is most marked in the lower lobes and is due to intrinsic fibrosis independent of the extent of the pleural fibrosis. There is an increase in collagen fibrous tissue which is most marked around the terminal bronchi and extends peripherally into the alveolar walls (Figs. 6 and 7). Coalescence leads to the obliteration of air spaces and the presence of isolated groups of alveolar cells. The rigidity and contraction of the lung tissue leads to widening of the distal bronchi and distorted rigid terminal airspaces lined with epithelium which is similar to bronchial epithelium but may be derived from transformation of the alveolar lining cells. This cystic or honeycomb lung is the end result of a change which occurs gradually but irregularly throughout the whole lung but is more marked in the lower lobes. Even at an early stage the fibrosis around the terminal bronchi spreading into the alveolar walls may disturb ventilation and gas exchange more than the radiological and pathological findings suggest (Schepers, 1965). Perivascular fibrosis may interfere with the distribution of blood to the alveoli and cause pulmonary hypertension (Bachirewa, 1968).

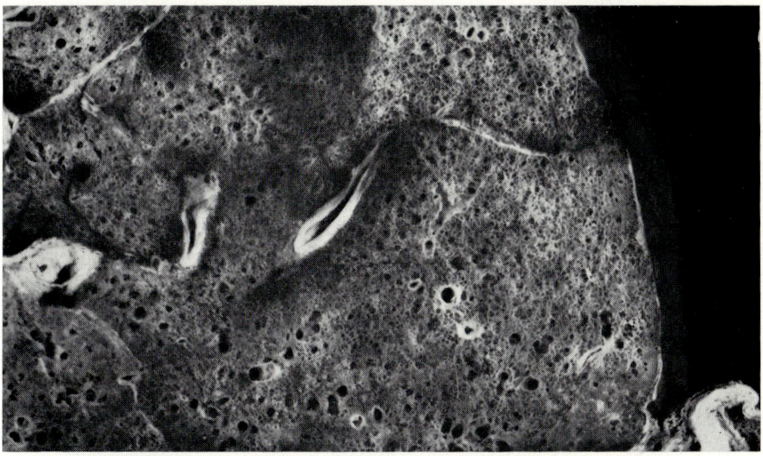

FIG. 7. Early peripheral fibrosis in the upper lobe of a man who had worked for many years as a pipe coverer but lived to the age of 86. Small areas of the lower lobes showed honeycomb change like Fig. 6 and part of a calcified pleural plaque is seen in the photograph.

The Pleura

Two changes are associated with exposure to asbestos, one affecting mainly the visceral and the other affecting mainly the parietal pleura.

(a) **Visceral Pleura.** This becomes involved by the diffuse fibrosis of the parenchyma already described and only becomes marked when the exposure is very heavy. Once the surface of the lung becomes immobile, adhesion to the parietal pleura develops and the space is obliterated.

(b) **Parietal Pleura.** Plaques form on the parietal pleura under circumstances which are not directly related to the pulmonary charges. They start as raised cartilaginous areas on the visceral surface of the ribs and the tendinous portion of the diaphragm. As they grow they may extend over the muscular part of the diaphragm and the intercostal spaces and

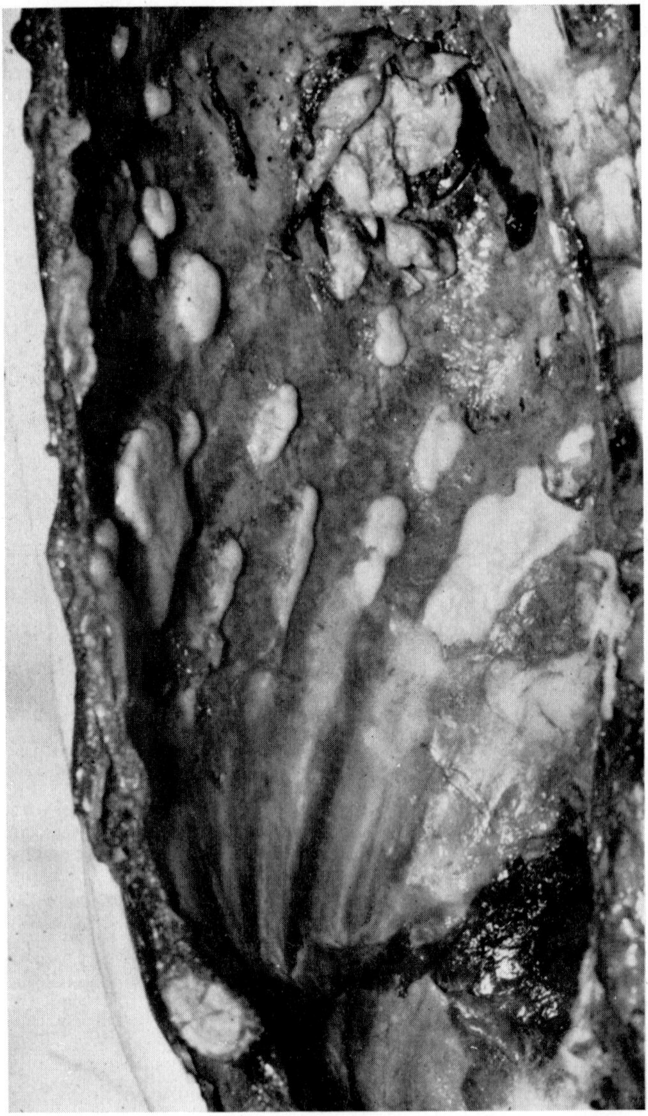

FIG. 8. Pleural Plaques.

(a) Chest wall from a painter who died of a localized mesothelioma at the age of 69. He had spent many years painting over the insulation in ship's engine rooms and later sanded down and painted asbestos "prefabs". The mesothelioma is seen on the upper part of the picture.

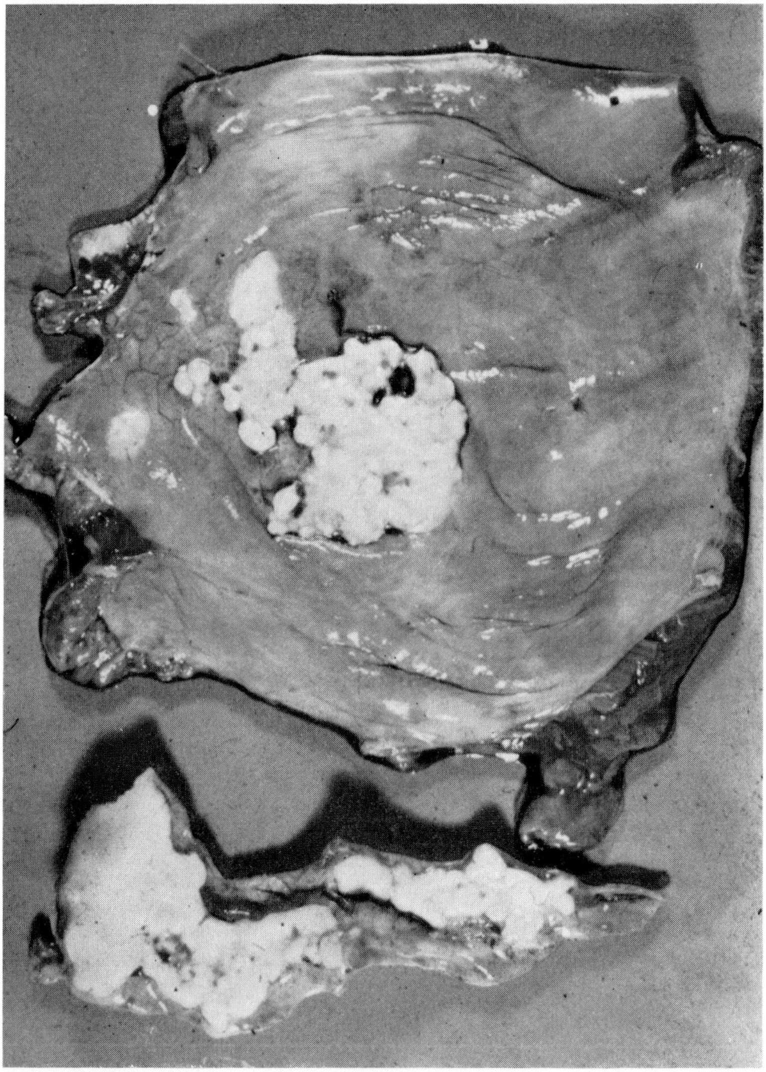

FIG. 8. Pleural Plaques.
(b) Diaphragm from a man of 76 who died of pulmonary fibrosis. He had worked as an asbestos storeman from 1919 to 1924 and again from 1940 to 1955.

coalesce with neighbouring lesions. They appear first and grow largest on the diaphragms, over the lower ribs posteriorly and the mid zone laterally and in front (Figs. 8a, b). They tend to coalesce along the paravertebral gutter and just lateral to the costochondral junctions.

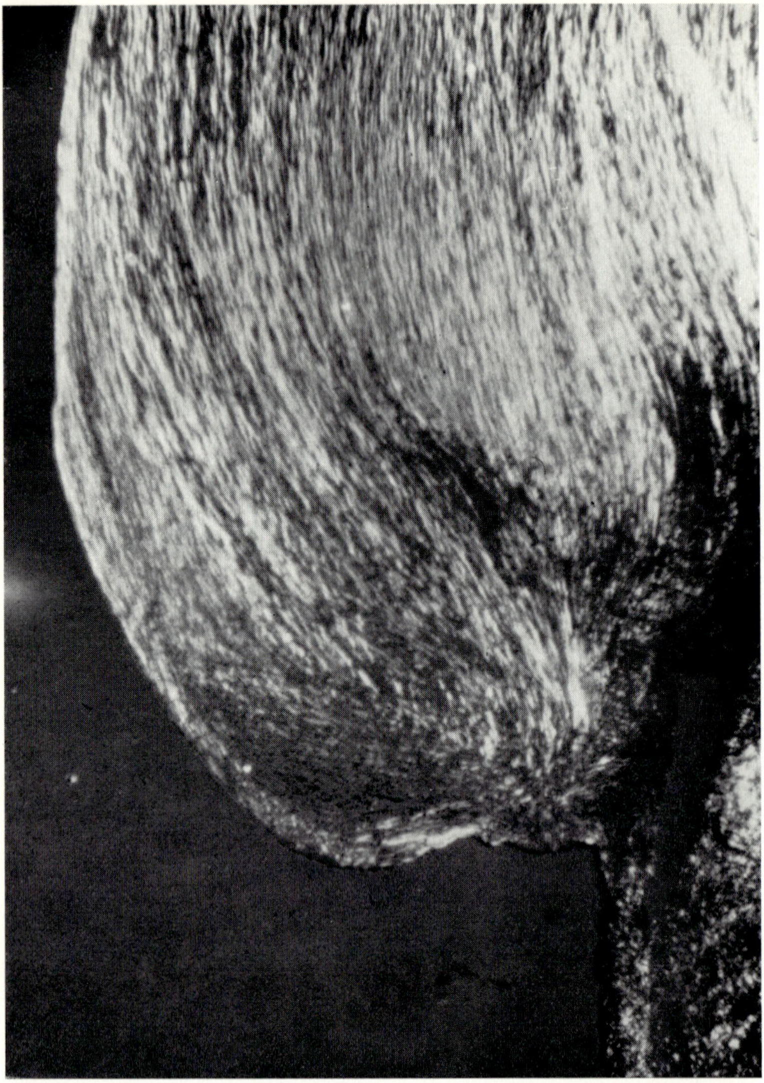

Fig. 9. Microscopic appearance of the edge of a pleural plaque in polarized light. Dense bundles of highly birefringent collagen lying between the elastic lamina and the serosal cells.

They occasionally appear on the pleural surface of the pericardium but never over the lung apices or in the costophrenic angles. They do not appear where the pleural space is obliterated by adhesions. Microscopically they consist of dense almost acellular collagen (Fig. 9) lying

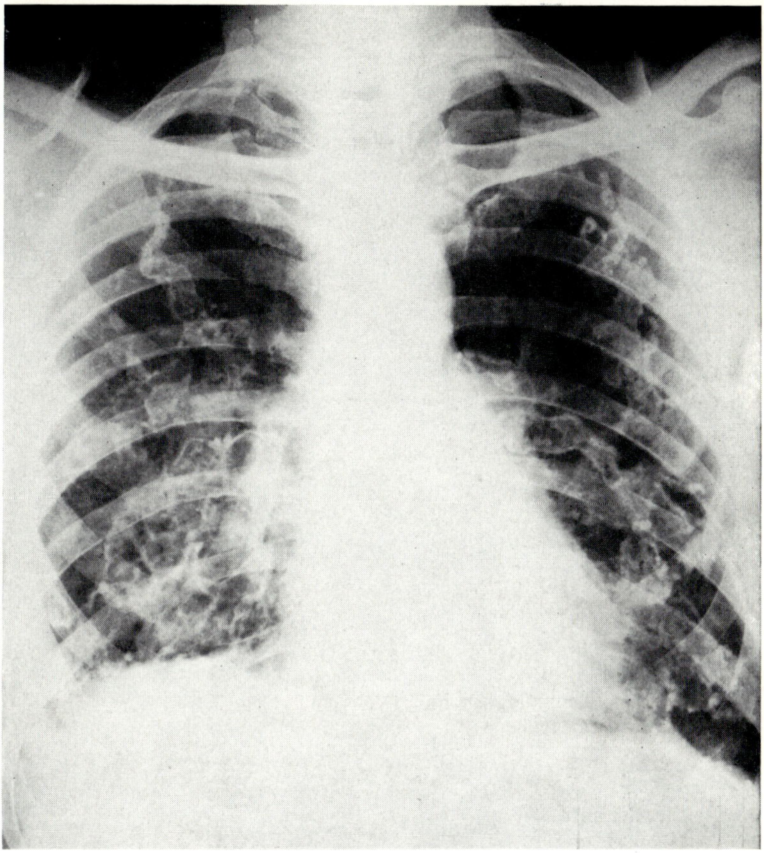

FIG. 10(a). Bilateral calcified pleural plaques. This man started as a pipe coverer and worked his way up to local manager in the insulation business. He died aged 63 of a mesothelioma the early signs of which are visible on the right side. (a) Whole chest. (b) Left upper zone.

between the elastic lamina and the serosal cells. In older people calcium is deposited near the pleural surface and the plaques become visible on X-ray.

Meurmann (1966) who has made an extensive study of these lesions in Finland relates them to occupational and environmental exposure to anthophyllite dust. Kiviluoto (1960) has suggested that asbestos fibres project from the pleural surface of the lung and cause the plaques in the parietal pleura by friction. Meurmann has described proliferative changes in the visceral pleura in patients with plaques but it is difficult to find asbestos in the lesions themselves.

Bilateral plaques with the typical radiological appearance (Fig. 10)

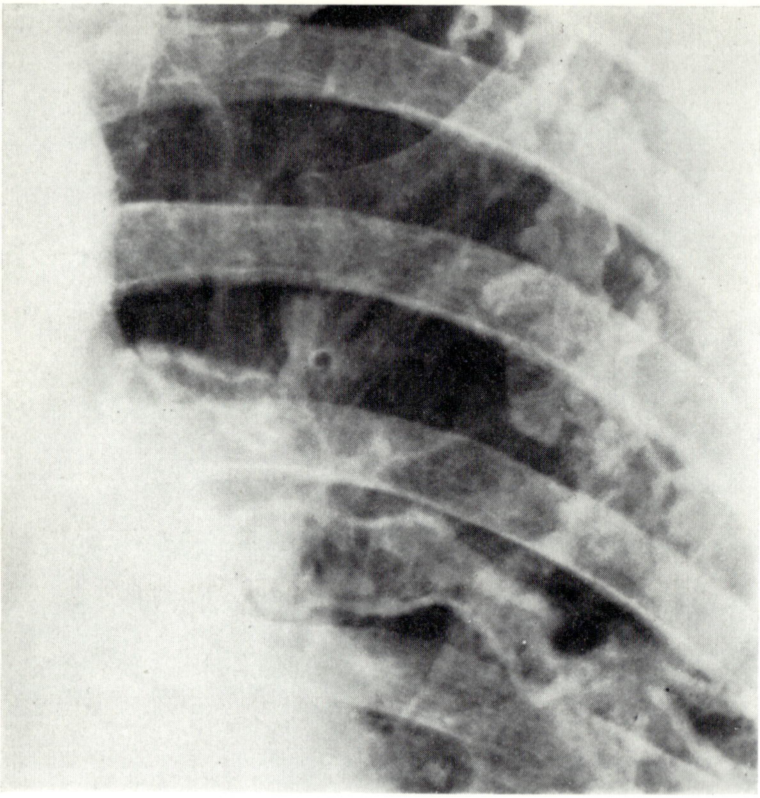

FIG. 10(b). (*Continued*).

seem to be characteristic of asbestos exposure. They are not associated with pulmonary fibrosis or malignancy in Finland. They are often associated with fibrosis and sometimes with malignancy in Britain where the exposure is mixed. They occur in some American groups exposed to chrysotile but not in others (Selikoff, 1965; Smith, 1966).

The Clinical Findings

Since 1930 the time course of asbestosis has been lengthened but the pattern of symptoms and signs of the disease has remained the same. The onset is insidious and in the early stages it is indistinguishable from any other chronic respiratory disease. Cough, with or without a little clear spit, is worse in winter than summer but not necessarily associated with acute respiratory episodes. Shortness of breath and a tightness or poorly localized pain in the chest appear relatively late by which time the fine basal rales and radiological changes, as well as definite dimunition in lung function, may be detected. The early detection of characteristic features of asbestosis which make the diagnosis certain in the individual cases is only possible in young and otherwise completely fit adults. The presence of asbestos warts on the hands and asbestos bodies in the sputum are evidence of exposure and are not related to the severity of pulmonary or pleural disease. But clubbing of the fingers occurs late and carries a strong probability of malignant change. In uncomplicated cases death usually follows a long period of severe respiratory incapacity with cyanosis and right-sided heart failure. But now that asbestosis develops more slowly patients live long enough to die of malignant disease rather than uncomplicated lung fibrosis.

Physiological Changes

The fibrotic changes in lung and pleura lead to a gradual reduction in total lung volume and vital capacity. This is not associated with any narrowing of the airways so that the forced expiratory volume and peak flow rates are relatively well maintained and the forced expiratory volume is often more than 80% of the vital capacity. This characteristic pattern is shared by other diffuse fibrotic lung diseases such as fibrosing alveolitis and sarcoidosis. As in these diseases there is interference with gas transfer. This can occur before there is recognizable radiological disease (Williams and Hugh Jones, 1960). But in practice the wide variation in the normal range make the single breath test of little value in the early case. More accurate evaluation of gas transfer by steady state methods at rest and on exercise may be of more diagnostic value but are too cumbersome for routine use.

None of these tests are very accurate when applied to individuals with early disease. This is partly because of the wide range of predicted normal values, but also because minimal airways disease (bronchitis or asthma) completely obscures the pattern. Bearing in mind that particularly in Britain most asbestos workers smoke and live in a heavily polluted atmosphere, these tests have little diagnostic value in men over the age of 45. However, if the workers concerned are tested at yearly or two-yearly intervals from the time of first employment, a much more precise diagnosis can be made. Even using the simplest ventilatory studies such as the vital capacity and forced expiratory volume the rate of fall off of these values with age is known with some precision. Having established the worker's normal value, plotting the serial changes against time will reveal deviation from normal at a much earlier stage.

Radiological Changes

The radiological changes which appear first in asbestosis depend upon the level of exposure. At the lowest level of exposure discrete pleural plaques and mesotheliomas may occur without lung changes. At intermediate levels of exposure such as now occurs in industry where there is good dust control, parenchymal and diffuse pleural changes only occur in an age group where other chronic lung disease and degenerative changes obscure the picture. The florid picture of diffuse lung and pleural damage which made the diagnosis of asbestosis on radiological grounds alone is now uncommon.

Pleural plaques are not detected in routine radiographs until they start to calcify which may take 15 to 20 years from first exposure. In a working population they are seldom present before the age of 45 unless there is a history of childhood exposure. The morphology of the calcification is characteristic in the advanced case because a continuous layer is deposited around the periphery of the plaque close to the pleural surface. The layer may be absent or too thin to show up in the central part of the plaque (Fig. 10). The presence of bilateral diaphragmatic and parietal plaques of the type illustrated is diagnostic of asbestos exposure. It must be distinguished from calcification in the fibrous residue of an empyema or a haemothorax. In neither instance does the calcification look the same, being more granular and dense in the centre of each pleural mass. Both can occasionally be bilateral but evidence of old tuberculous pulmonary disease, drainage scars or fractured ribs suggest the correct diagnosis. Clinical history can help but it is surprising how difficult it is to get a clear history as to the nature of a chest illness which may have occurred 20–30 years previously.

Diffuse Pleural Changes. The radiological changes depend both upon the subpleural fibrosis of the lung parenchyma and upon the tendency for the two layers of the pleura to become adherent. Unlike the plaques these changes affect the visceral rather than the parietal pleura until adhesion occurs. Initially there is a loss of the smooth inner surface of the pleura so that the surface of the diaphragm and the pericardium has a blurred appearance. The fissures become thickened and more easily indentified.

Obliteration of the costophrenic angle, irregular peaking of the diaphragm and a definite thickening of the pleura against the lower part of the chest wall and over the lung apices usually occur later. These changes are seldom seen without obvious parenchymal disease. At this stage it is often possible to see that the parenchymal shadows run into the thickened pleura and are part of the same process.

Parenchymal Changes. It is important to look for evidence of fibrous tissue within the lung substance and for the distortion of the lung caused by the pleural and intrapulmonary fibrosis.

In spite of the even distribution of inhaled asbestos fibres throughout the lung (Bell and Elmes, 1968), the changes are first seen in the lower zones. This effect is only in part due to the greater thickness of lung penetrated by the X-ray beam, because there is a relative contraction of the lower lobes. The oblique fissure moves backwards and downwards and the diaphragm rises as the volume occupied by the lower lobe is

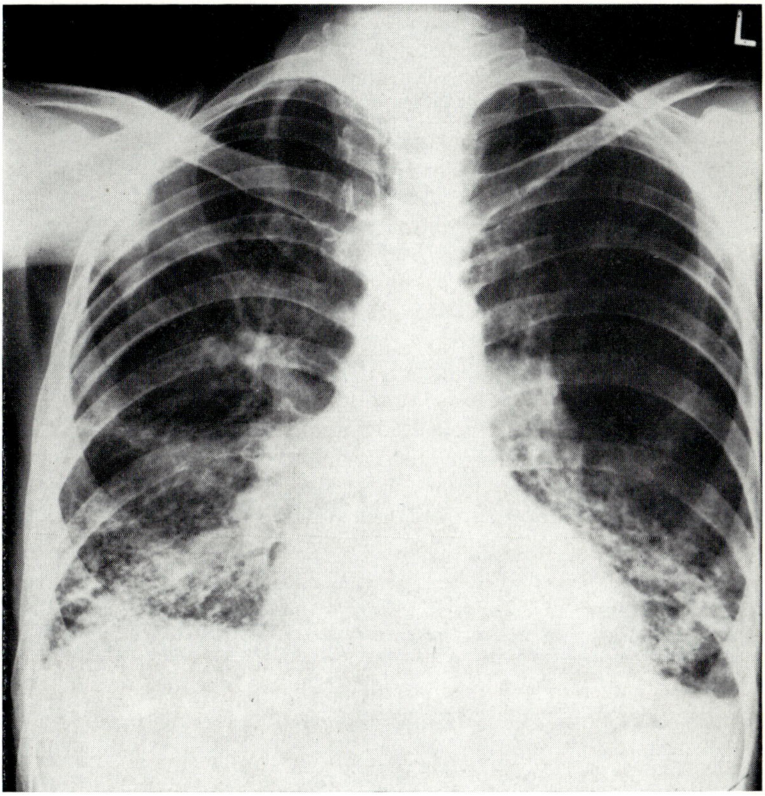

FIG. 11. It is not possible to reproduce for printing the early radiological changes in the lung parenchyma. This man worked as a pipe coverer from 1935 until he was disabled by asbestosis in 1960. He died in 1963 of an adenocarcinoma of the caecum at the age of 54. This is an unusually severe asbestosis for a pipe coverer of this age, showing marked bilateral basal fibrosis with honeycomb appearance.

restricted. Within the lower lobes the bronchi and vessels become crowded together and the distal ends curve backwards (the "birch broom" appearance) (Bohlig, 1964). This appearance shows well on bronchogram and angiogram but as the parenchyma fibrosis increases it is apparent on ordinary X-ray. The presence of tubular bronchiectasis and honeycomb change may also become obvious without special techniques (Fig. 11).

These changes are non-specific and may be difficult to distinguish from chronic inflammatory changes especially in the older bronchitic patient. But symmetry and association with the pleural changes may make a positive diagnosis of asbestosis possible in relatively young heavily exposed men. The distribution of the fibrosis around the peripheral bronchi and running out into the pleura gives rise to patterns of shadowing in the periphery which may look like small discrete opacities of the various types which have been used in the international classification of other pneumoconioses. However, the appearances are not clear cut and some regard as characteristic a band-like appearance which has been likened to the pattern produced by X-raying crumpled strips of aluminium foil (Bohlig, 1965). The precise picture may vary between occupational groups and be as much dependent on the character of the other dusts inhaled and the extent of cigarette smoking, bronchitis, etc. It is perhaps for this reason that it has taken so long to reach an international agreement on how to record the radiological findings in asbestos workers (Elmes, 1971). It is also for this reason that the diagnosis of early asbestosis in the individual can seldom be based on these changes alone although in epidemiological studies of large groups radiology may be more sensitive than physiological tests.

In the study of any group of asbestos workers there is a noticeable lack of correlation between the extent of exposure and the amount of radiological change in individuals. There is a relatively high frequency of abnormal titres to rheumatoid factor (Pernis, Vigliani, and Selikoff, 1965) and antinuclear factor (Turner-Warwick, 1970) in asbestos workers with marked radiological evidence of parenchymal disease. But it is not clear whether the autoimmune abnormality is due to, or the cause of, the dust lung lesions. Nor is there any evidence that the autoimmune response modifies the radiological pattern of parenchymal lung damage.

Criteria for the Diagnosis of Asbestosis

In the study of groups of men on a prospective basis the detection of a significant hazard may be the result of any of a number of serial observations. The criteria for diagnosis in the individual, either for the purposes of advising him to change occupation, or in the support of claims for industrial injury or compensation, are arbitrary and based on four kinds of evidence. The pneumoconiosis panels have established such criteria which they apply to each individual claim. If the evidence is sufficient to satisfy one of these panels, then a civil court will also be satisfied. But the ultimate proof rests on the histological changes in the lungs. Biopsy by current methods is not sufficiently safe to be used for legal purposes alone and therefore ultimate proof may have to wait until autopsy.

The four kinds of evidence to be considered are—

(1) Evidence of Exposure. This can occur in the home or environment, but it is now extremely rare for exposure to be sufficient to cause asbestosis unless it occurs for several hours most working days. Although evidence of fibrosis can occur in under ten years, it is unusual for conditions to be bad enough now to cause detectable changes in under 20 years. The presence of asbestos fibres in the spit is evidence of current exposure and of asbestos bodies of past exposure. Neither is evidence of lung damage.

(2) Clinical Evidence of restrictive lung disease. The slow increase in breathlessness and tightness in the chest can be difficult to distinguish from bronchitis on the one hand and angina pectoris on the other. Although productive cough is usually present it is a relatively minor feature. Compared with angina the tightness hasn't the characteristic radiation or response to trinitrin. Fine basal rales are only heard when disability is severe. Asbestos warts indicate exposure but not pulmonary disease. Clubbing occurs late and may indicate malignancy.

(3) Radiological Evidence. Pleural plaques are evidence of exposure but do not indicate disease. Diffuse lung and pleural changes as described above, with evidence of contraction of the lower lobes, are strongly suggestive of asbestosis but can be due to other fibrotic lung disease.

(4) Physiological Evidence. Reduced lung volumes and transfer factor coupled with normal airways resistance indicate asbestosis or other fibrotic lung disease.

Next, sarcoidosis or other systemic disease which might cause a similar picture must be excluded by clinical and laboratory investigations. This leaves fibrosing alveolitis and similar primary lung diseases which are so rare that in the presence of definite exposure a diagnosis of asbestosis can be made on probability.

Carcinoma of the Lung

The collection of data which resulted from the 1932 regulations led to the discovery of another more sinister hazard. Up to 1935 the recorded causes of death in men certified as having asbestosis included 7% with primary cancer of the lung. This rose to 17% in 1947 (Merewether, 1949) and to 54% in 1965 (Buchanan, 1965). Cases had been described before 1948 but this was the first proof of the association. Many other studies have confirmed it since.

Because of the long interval between first exposure and the development of cancer, it was hoped that the cases being observed were the result of high exposure in factories before the regulations came into force. The possibility that the regulations had eliminated the hazard was strengthened by studies on workers in a Rochdale asbestos factory (Knox, Holmes, Doll and Hill, 1968):

Cancer of the Lung in Male Factory Workers up to 1961

Total exposure	Exposure before 1933	Deaths Observed	Deaths Expected
Over 20 years	Over 10 years	12	1·18
,,	Less than 10 years	5	1·57
,,	None	2	1·35

In this factory dust suppression has been so effective that not only are workers starting employment since 1933 unlikely to get asbestosis, but as yet they seem no more likely to develop cancer of the lung than other men. The factory does not appear to be typical of working conditions with asbestos in the British Isles as a whole because of the steady rise in the number of cases of asbestosis certified each year and the proportion found to have lung cancer when they die (Buchanan, 1965). The average age at death due to uncomplicated asbestosis in Britain has risen from 49 years in 1940 to 60 years in 1960–3, but average age at death due to lung cancer has remained at about 56 years. Therefore, although the general level of asbestos exposure has fallen, it has not fallen sufficiently to eliminate the risk of cancer of the lung.

The number of new certified cases of asbestosis has risen from 17 in 1950 to 67 in 1963 (McVittie, 1965). Some of this is due to an increase of cases from factories covered by the 1931 regulations. But between 1963 and 1965, 52% of the new cases arose from occupations not covered by the original regulations. Most of these were insulation workers and failure to include these men in the schedule requiring medical supervision has had serious consequences. In a retrospective study of all the insulation workers who were employed in Belfast in 1940 it has been shown that these men were at risk to asbestosis and, more seriously, to lung cancer. The mortality experience of this group of men has been compared with the rest of the male population and it is apparent that they were already dying prematurely by 1950 (Figs. 12 and 13) and over the whole period the average age at death was only 55 years (Elmes and Simpson, 1968). Most of this excessive mortality was due to cancer of the lung and pleura (Fig. 14), but there was also an excess of deaths due to chronic non-malignant lung disease and due to other cancers. Similar results have been obtained with insulation workers in New York (Hammond, Selikoff and Churg, 1965) and the indications are that exposure is comparable to two groups of American asbestos factory workers (Enterline, 1965; Mancuso and El-Attar, 1968). In these American studies gastrointestinal neoplasms account for most of the cases of non-respiratory cancers. But the Rochdale factory study does not show an excess of other cancers and although they are described from a factory in East London (Smither, 1965), it is not clear whether the frequency is in excess of expected. Further work is necessary to

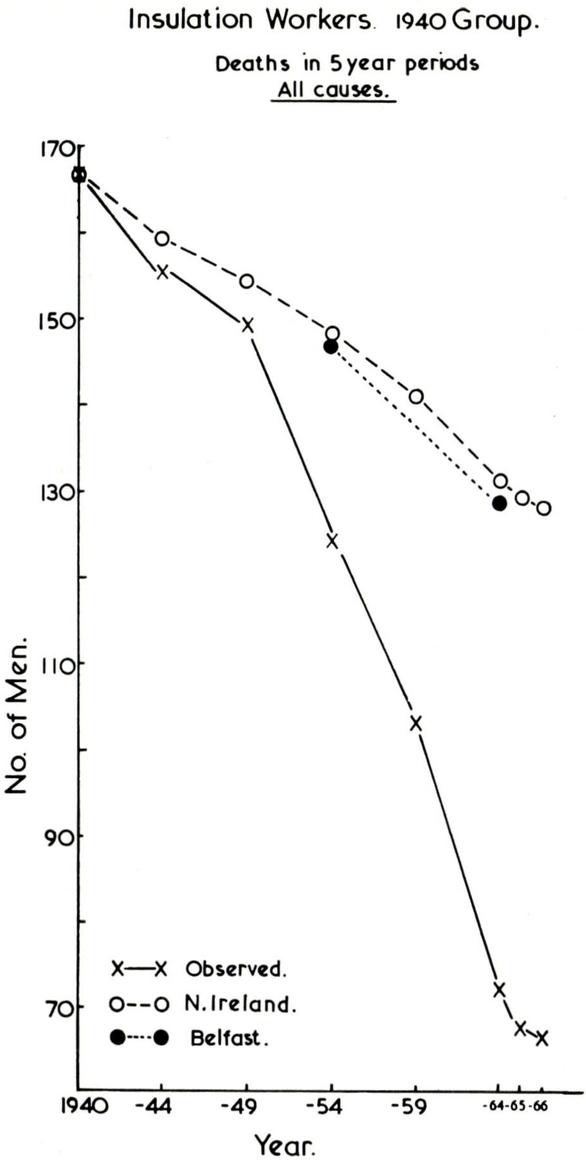

FIG. 12. Cumulative mortality experience of pipe coverers who were employed in 1940, compared with the general population of N. Ireland and of Belfast City. Matched for age and sex. All causes.

determine whether these other cancers, particularly those of the gastrointestinal tract, really are of importance in some or all types of asbestos exposure. There is evidence (Newhouse and Wagner, 1969) that some of the excess cases of "gastrointestinal cancer" observed may be due to failure to recognize peritoneal mesotheliomas.

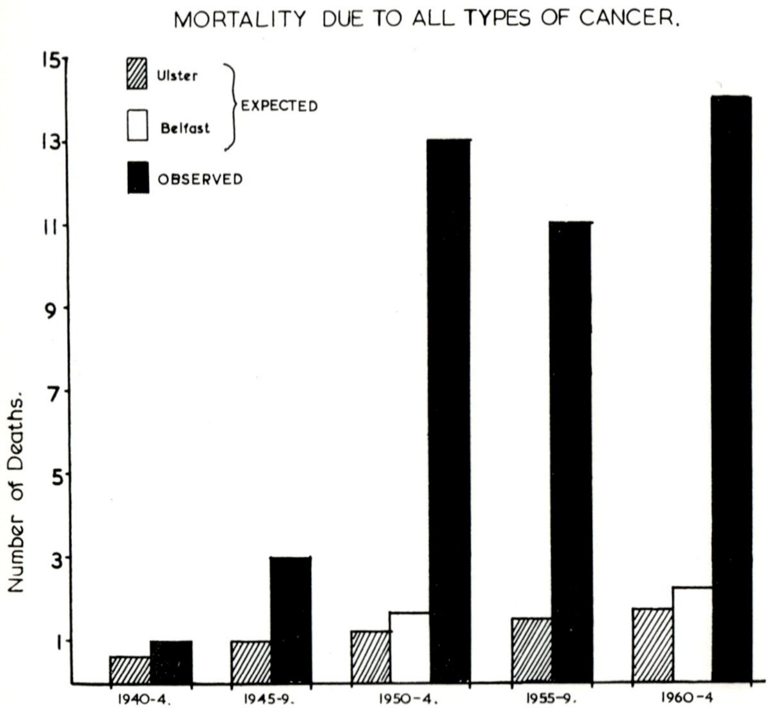

FIG. 13. All types of cancer. Mortality experience amongst pipe coverers who were employed in 1940. 5-year periods, matched for age and sex with the general population of Ulster and Belfast.

Cancer of the lung in asbestos workers shows a similar pattern to lung cancer occurring in the population as a whole. The peak age at death is between 50 and 60 years and there is evidence (Selikoff, Churg, Hammond and Kaffenburgh, 1968) that the effect of smoking is more than simply additive. In most series from Britain there are too few non-smokers to draw statistically valid conclusions nor can the relevance of atmospheric pollution be assessed. Some series show a predominance of lower lobe cancers (Bohlig and Jacob, 1956; Hourihane and McCaughey, 1966), but all three histological types are involved. In women adenocarcinomas predominate but again this may be due to the ancillary effect of more smoking in men inducing more squamous and oat celled carcinoma.

The prognosis of cancer of the lung in asbestos workers is even worse than it is in the general population because the pulmonary fibrosis and obliteration of the pleura makes operation technically more difficult. It has also been suggested (Swinburne, 1968) that in the presence of asbestosis there is a tendency towards early pleural involvement and a mesothelioma-like spread of any pulmonary neoplasm. Postoperatively the remaining fibrosed lung is less able to compensate for the loss of functioning tissue.

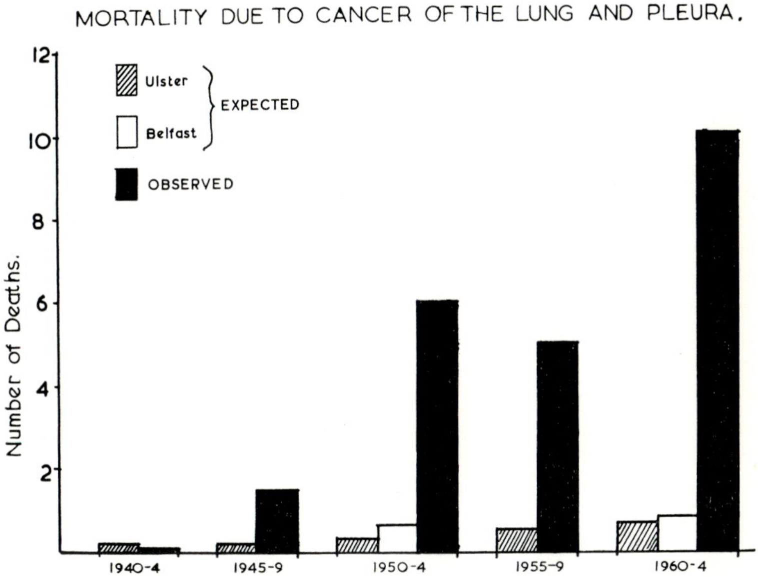

FIG. 14. Cancer of the lung and pleura. Mortality experience amongst pipe coverers who were employed in 1940. 5-year periods, matched for age and sex with the general population of Ulster and Belfast.

Mesotheliomas of the Pleura and Peritoneum

Pathology. Malignant mesothelial tumours of the pleura had been described by Stout and Murray in 1942, but many pathologists found it difficult to differentiate these rather pleomorphic tumours from the metastases of other primary tumours. McCaughey (1958) described 15 diffuse pleural mesothelial tumours and demonstrated the way in which the pattern was made up of two cell elements. (1) The fibrous element, which varies from a picture resembling a spindle celled sarcoma right through to dense almost acellular tissue resembling the scarring left by chronic inflammation. (2) The tubular or endothelial element: these cuboidal or spheroidal cells may occur in small groups in clefts in the fibrous tissue or may line spaces to resemble renal tubular epithelium. Larger spaces may be filled with tubulo-papillary patterns merging into solid masses with a scanty fibrous stroma. A single tumour may show these variations of both tissue elements from area to area so that a small biopsy may be very misleading.

In the early stages the tumour is often associated with the effusion of fluid, which usually contains large quantities of hyaluronic acid (Wagner, Munday and Harington, 1962); it may also contain blood. The fluid lies free in the pleura or peritoneum and may contain cells which an experienced exfoliative cytologist can recognize as arising from a malignant mesothelioma so that a presumptive diagnosis of diffuse mesothelioma can sometimes be made. As the tumour spreads over the surface of the visceral and parietal pleura or peritoneum the space becomes loculated and very often obliterated. At the same time movement both of the parieties and viscera becomes progressively restricted. Limited local invasion occurs sometimes giving rise to pain because of the invasion of bone and nerve. But rapid invasion of the local tissues seldom occurs except after damage by surgery or radiation. The absolute diagnosis of mesothelioma is made on observing this pattern of growth at postmortem and on eliminating other sources of malignancy (Fig. 15). The presence of some regional lymph node involvement and occasional haematogenous metastases has been accepted as compatible with the diagnosis provided the other features are typical. Since the association with asbestos exposure has been established, the presence of asbestos bodies in the lungs, with or without associated fibrosis, has been taken as supporting evidence for the diagnosis of diffuse mesothelioma.

Recognition of Diffuse Mesotheliomas and their Association with Asbestos

At about the same time as McCaughey (1958) was describing mesotheliomas as a pathological entity, a group of patients with malignant pleural effusions were being investigated in South Africa. The autopsy findings were similar to McCaughey's cases but the synchronous appearance of a number of cases in one district suggested an environmental cause. Wagner and his colleagues (Wagner, Sleggs and Marchand, 1960) could only find one common factor, environmental exposure to crocidolite, in this group of patients.

Both clinicians and pathologists began searching for similar cases and by the end of 1964 there were 170 histologically proven cases in South Africa and 240 cases in Britain. Many of them were discovered by reappraisal of cases coming to autopsy in the previous 10 or 15 years. But unless a large number of cases have been missed entirely, there appears to have been a rapid increase in the incidence of this kind of tumour.

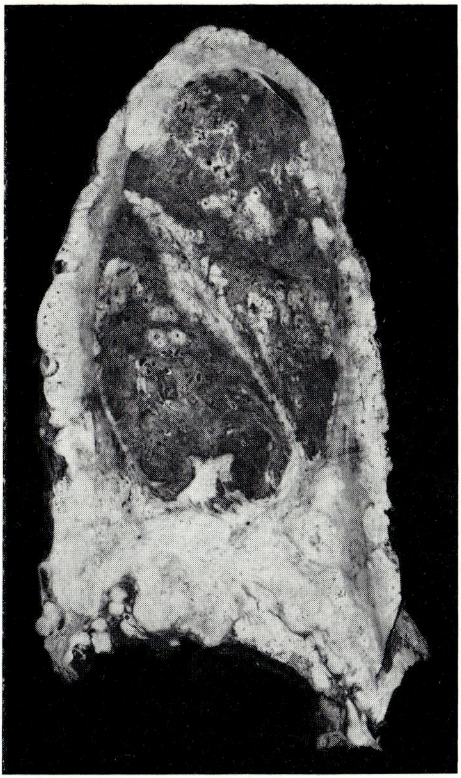

FIG. 15. Typical postmortem appearance of mesothelioma of the pleura in a 62-year-old man who had worked in the shipyard for 31 years first as a driller's and then a plater's helper with only casual exposure to asbestos. The lung is compressed with areas of suppurating bronchopneumonia. The tumour consists of bands of dense fibrous tissue with patches of more cellular tissue tending to grow outwards rather than invade the lung. The diaphragm is replaced by tumour. On histology the lung showed scanty asbestos bodies and no fibrosis.

The evidence that these tumours are related to asbestos exposure has been collected in various ways—

(a) Asbestos bodies in the lung. Whenever lung tissue has been searched for bodies an association has been noted. In one series there were bodies present in 80% of cases of mesothelioma but in only 20% of the control population (Elmes and Wade, 1965). There are always some cases where no asbestos bodies can be found, but it is known that a lung containing a few bodies may contain many asbestos fibres. Depending upon what method is used for examining the lungs asbestos bodies may be found in from 20 to 50% of the lungs of the inhabitants of large cities (Thompson, 1965). The inhabitants of small town and country areas show correspondingly less evidence of environmental exposure (Ashcroft, 1968). The surprising result of this type of investigation was the widespread evidence of inhaled asbestos in the general population at a level approaching that thought to be important in causing mesotheliomas. Evidence of lung fibrosis such as is seen in asbestosis did not seem to be essential in the pathogenesis of mesothelioma.

(b) Exposure to asbestos. Two types of study revealed this association. In one a population of asbestos workers was followed up and cases of mesothelioma discovered far in excess of the general population (Hammond, Selikoff and Churg, 1965; Enticknap and Smither, 1964). But this failed to account for all the cases occurring in a community. By the other method the past occupations of all patients dying with mesothelioma are studied. This has revealed that in many cases the exposure was not due to regular work with asbestos. In one series (Elmes and Wade, 1965) only a quarter of the cases had used asbestos regularly in their work. In about the same number of cases there was no history of exposure at all. The rest of the Belfast cases had occasionally been exposed to asbestos at work. Owen (1964) found a similar distribution in another shipbuilding port, Liverpool. In London (Newhouse and Thompson, 1965) and South Africa (Wagner, Sleggs and Marchand, 1960), numerous cases of environmental exposure have been reported. These were due to dust produced by mines and factories contaminating the neighbouring atmosphere or being brought home on working clothes and affecting other members of the family.

Two important facts have emerged from this type of study:

(a) The exposure may be quite brief and the interval between first exposure very long. Children playing on the waste heaps of asbestos mines may develop mesotheliomas in the third or fourth decade (Wagner *et al.*, 1960), but when the exposure is occupational the average interval may be 40 years and the mean age at death over 60 years (Elmes and Wade, 1965). The brevity of exposure and long intervals make the proof of the relationship between exposure and tumour especially difficult, and prevention even more difficult.

(b) Not all asbestos mines, factories or occupations seem to be associated with mesothelioma. Many of the industries and mining areas are too new or have too transient a population to be sure of their safety. At the present time mesotheliomas have been proven in association with the mining of crocidolite in Africa and

Western Australia but not with the mining of chrysotile or amosite in Africa. A few mesotheliomas have been recorded in the Canadian asbestos mining towns but some milling of imported fibre has occurred there (Cartier, 1955). No mesotheliomas have been reported from the Finnish anthophyllite mines or from the chrysotile mines in Russia or Cyprus. Mesotheliomas have been reported from most of the user industry countries such as Germany, Sweden, Britain, Canada and the United States. When individual factories or occupational groups in Britain are studied, the distribution is very uneven. Most of the London cases have been traced back to a firm which has always used crocidolite. The insulation workers in the shipbuilding industry, particularly those doing limpet spraying have also used crocidolite from time to time and here mesotheliomas have always been found when they have been searched for. But only 5 mesotheliomas have been detected in Rochdale where the factory has only used small quantities of crocidolite. No mesotheliomas have so far been found near Cleckheaton where crocidolite is not normally used. The evidence suggesting that crocidolite is the only cause of human mesothelioma is circumstantial but very strong. Experiments have shown, however, that amosite and chrysotile can also cause mesothelial tumours in rats when administered by intrapleural inoculation (Wagner, 1968).

Clinical Picture

The tumour is slow growing and the onset of symptoms correspondingly insidious. A dull ache in the affected side of the chest or in the abdomen may be present for weeks or months before the patient seeks medical advice and before there is any definite disability or abnormality on examination. Rapidly increasing breathlessness or abdominal distention may then occur as effusion develops and occasionally is not preceded by any other symptoms. The effusion may be clear and viscous containing both hyaluronic acid and recognizable mesothelioma cells. But it is often not of diagnostic value especially when it is heavily blood-stained. Wasting and weakness occur late and the pain may become more severe if the nerves in the chest or abdominal wall become infiltrated. In the pleural cases there is progressive immobilization of that side of the chest with constriction of the lung and a shift of the mediastinum to that side when the effusion is absorbed or is removed (Fig. 16). In the peritoneal cases abdominal pain and alternating diarrhoea and constipation presage intestinal obstruction. Hard confluent masses may become palpable. The disease usually runs a 1- to 2-year course from the onset of symptoms and terminally both pleural cavities, pericardium and peritoneum may be involved by direct extension so that the primary site may be difficult to determine.

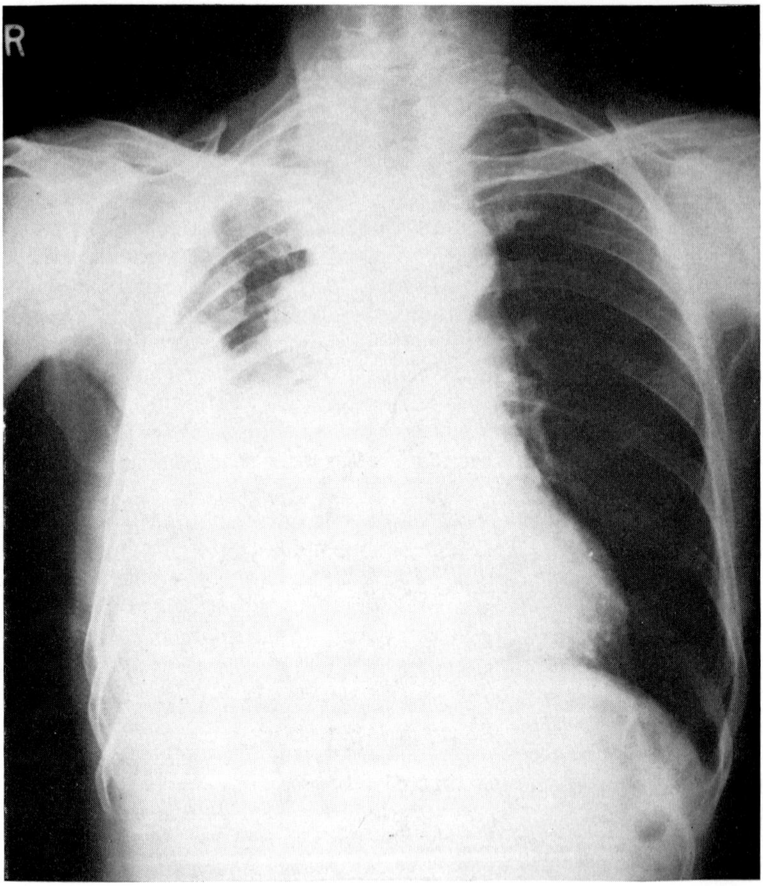

FIG. 16. Typical radiological appearance of mesothelioma. Note the irregular tumour mass in the pleura space and the absence of other evidence of asbestos exposure. The mass in the upper mediastinum was direct extension and not lymphnode spread. The tumour had extended through the diaphragm and seeded over the peritoneum which contained two litres of fluid at postmortem. This man died at the age of 62 in 1966 and had worked as an apprentice plumber from 1918–24. He did various types of plumbing work in ships from 1940–64. He had contact with but never worked continuously with asbestos in either period.

The prognosis is not improved by radiotherapy, cytotoxic drugs or attempts at excision. But it is sometimes of symptomatic value to delay the reaccumulation of fluid in either pleura or peritoneum by the injection of nitrogen mustard. Biopsy, either by needle or open operation, may cause the growth to fungate through the skin. As the precise diagnosis does not help in treatment it is probably better to wait for an autopsy rather than risk this distressing complication.

Prevention of Hazards due to Asbestos

1. **Asbestosis in factories.** The application of the 1931 regulations in Britain has made it possible to correlate morbidity and mortality with levels of dust exposure in the factories over the years. The British Occupational Hygiene Society has published *Hygiene Standards for Chrysotile Asbestos Dust* (Roach, 1968a) which is based on such a study. In a factory which uses mainly chrysotile it has been shown that the frequency of clinical asbestosis before the retiring age is related to the product of the concentration of dust and the duration exposure. In this factory less than 1% of the men develop asbestosis provided they are exposed to less than 100 fibre years/cm^3* during their working career. This seems to be true whether the exposure is 4 fibres/cm^3 for 25 years or 10 fibres per cm^3 for 10 years, but the groups were studied over relatively long periods so that the rule may not apply to brief exposure to very high dust concentrations. The Hygiene Society recommend a maximum lifetime exposure of 100 fibre years/cm^3. The fibre concentrations are based on a membrane filter method counting particles over 5 μ in length and at least 3 times as long as they are thick. This means that whole dust levels up to 1·9 fibres/cm^3 are tolerable, the Society recommends that if the level cannot be brought down to this, masks must be worn. Where exposure to over 50 fibres/cm^3 is unavoidable a pressure-fed breathing apparatus must be used even for short periods.

This standard is more stringent than that resulting from the United States Public Health Survey of 1938. But if applied to chrysotile it should bring down asbestosis to under 1% and eliminate the added hazard of lung cancer (Roach).

The difficulty is that this standard is expensive to achieve even under factory conditions and may not apply to the other types of asbestos or asbestos mixed with other materials. The cost is indicated by the fact that in a large textile factory the cost of dust suppression represents 2·7% of the total manufacturing costs (Hills, 1965). Maintenance of dust suppression equipment can be hazardous to the engineers, and for this reason settling chambers have been replaced by filter systems. Even if dust-laden air is no longer blown out into the neighbourhood, the material removed by filters must still be disposed of safely.

2. **Asbestosis in user industries.** Asbestos products used in the factory manufacture of consumer goods should present no real problem provided the workers and the management are aware that a hazard exists. The machining and sawing of cement and plastic materials reinforced with asbestos creates an obvious hazard which can be treated in the same way as the processes in the asbestos cement or textile factory.

* fibre years/cm^3 = Average concentration of dust in fibres/cm^3 × no. of yrs. exposure.

It is possible to segregate all "on site" drilling, sawing and other preparation work. Factory methods of dust control can be applied to this area; all workmen who have to be in this area can wear masks and wear protective clothing; all other workmen can be excluded. But, in spite of prefabrication, there will still remain some dust production where the asbestos material is actually used or when it is being dismantled. Again masks and protective clothing can be used and other workmen must be kept away. A typical example of this hazard is the dismantling of insulation during the repair or demolition of ships. This is an extremely dusty procedure, carried out in confined spaces, very often with the ship's ventilation system not working. Harries (1968) has devised a complete scheme for the protection of workers in Naval Dockyards and Naval contract work which includes the provision of pressurized hoods for the insulation of workers, the sealing of debris in airtight bags and the rigid exclusion of other workmen.

To achieve acceptance of these measures in the rest of the shipbuilding and constructional industry may prove difficult. The workers dislike the bother and discomfort of the hoods, masks and protective clothing. The employers dislike not only the cost of providing equipment but also the delays caused by the shortening of the working shift and the necessity for excluding other workers. Work flow planning becomes more complex and contract dates more difficult to achieve. However, the hazard for insulation workers has been well enough documented and is known to the insulation workers. Realization by others will come in time and entry into hazardous work will dwindle unless protective measures are taken.

The hazard must exist in many other occupations but has not been assessed. When it is appreciated by both employer and working man that asbestos dust is always a potential hazard then precautions will be taken and tolerated.

3. **Cancer of the lung.** The "standard" may protect chrysotile asbestos factory workers against cancer. But no such accurate figures exist for the other types of asbestos in factory use. There are, however, some indications that the association between exposure to asbestos and lung cancer does only occur when there is an appreciable incidence of asbestosis. In the two studies of insulation workers the two conditions co-exist (Elmes and Simpson, 1968; Selikoff *et al.*, 1968). In the factory using crocidolite mixed with other asbestos fibres (Smither, 1965), cancer of the lung was found in about one-third of the deaths at a time when 2–3% of the labour force were being certified as new cases of asbestosis each year. The association between smoking and cancer of the lung in asbestos workers has already been mentioned. At the present time it is probable that the application of the "Hygiene Standard for Chrysolite dust" to all asbestos fibres may remove the hazard of

bronchial cancer as well. But it would also seem prudent to warn all workers that cigarette smoking may materially increase the risk.

4. **Mesotheliomas and other forms of malignancy.** Although there may be an increased frequency of death due to malignant disease other than cancer of the lung, evidence in relation to levels of exposure is less satisfactory. So far an increase in cancers of the gastro-intestinal tract and possibly the genito-urinary tract have only been observed on the groups already known to have an appreciable incidence of lung fibrosis and lung cancer. No studies have been made of miscellaneous cancer in low exposure groups.

In the case of mesothelioma the situation is different in that in a large proportion of cases the exposure to asbestos has only been discovered in retrospect. The apparently brief and trivial levels of exposure seem to indicate that only complete exclusion of the fibres responsible can prevent this disease. The evidence so far indicates that crocidolite may be the only cause of mesothelioma and it seems reasonable to stop using this fibre except under careful supervision. If this fibre is the only form of asbestos that can be used for a specific purpose, then it must be handled in such a way that there is no danger of dust inhalation. The crocidolite should be labelled clearly as dangerous at all stages of manufacture and probably the finished product should also carry a warning label. Asbestos incorporated in pitch and similar material to make battery cases and roofing felt may seem safe forever until it is remembered what may happen when this material is burnt on the rubbish tip on the windward side of a town.

Regulations. Government regulations with regard to the control of this sort of hazard have two basic defects. The Government is unwilling to impose regulations on any industrial process until it has been proven hazardous. Secondly, the Government is unwilling to compel workers to undergo periodic medical examination unless this enables the worker to withdraw from hazardous employment before the point where the damage to his health is irreversible. Unfortunately the application of these two principles to asbestos hazards is particularly inappropriate.

(1) Asbestos is already used in a large number of processes which have not yet been proven to be hazardous. New processes are continually being devised and adopted.

(2) Existing medical information about the dust levels and type of fibre in relation to both cancer of the lung and other organs and in particular about mesotheliomas is incomplete. Therefore, it is not possible to predict from chemical analysis or from dust counts whether any particular process is hazardous or not.

The situation is made more difficult by the time course of the illnesses:

(a) A man may have an apparently normal chest X-ray and lung function tests after 30 years in a job with constant exposure and still develop serious asbestosis before he dies;

(b) The average age at death from cancer of the lung in asbestos workers is between 50 and 60 years irrespective of the age at which they were first exposed;

(c) Mesotheliomas occur on the average 40 years after first exposure at work even when the exposure has been brief. These tumours often develop after the worker has retired.

Therefore it is not possible to tell whether an occupation is hazardous unless the workers concerned are followed until they die. This means that in order to discover whether an occupation is hazardous all workers must be registered and the causes of death analysed as part of the routine surveyance.

Periodic examination (clinical, radiological or physiological) are of little value to the individual worker because they do not:

(a) enable the man to stop work before irreversible changes are present. Indeed as in the more severe degrees of silicosis the lung fibrosis tends to progress after exposure has ceased;

(b) periodic examination might permit the diagnosis of cancer a little earlier than would normally occur but would not change the prognosis.

Whereas registration followed by analysis of causes of death is the ultimate check as to the efficiency of the precautions taken against such a hazard as asbestos, it is a very slow method. The quickest method of checking whether precautions are effective is by periodic medical examination. As soon as physiological evidence of asbestosis appears in a group of workers, then this indicates a hazardous level of exposure even to the safer forms of asbestos. This may precede death or evidence of malignant disease by 15 or more years and this period of time is therefore saved and a large number of new workers who would have done this work in the future can be protected.

Summary

Asbestos is a fibrous mineral silicate with a wide variety of industrial uses. Its popularity for both manufacturers and users is based on its high resistance to heat and chemicals, its great strength and the fact that it is relatively easy to mine and process in large quantities. It is, therefore, cheap.

Because it is comparatively inert and indestructible, it persists in the environment and has been in widespread use for so long that the majority of the population have contact with it at some time in their lives. A careful search of the lungs of people dying in cities has revealed asbestos in over half the individuals. Except in areas where asbestos is mined or is present in the soil, country dweller's lungs contain less asbestos.

But the manufacturers and public as a whole were so impressed by the inert nature of asbestos that the medical evidence was virtually ignored until Merewether and Price's investigation in 1930. One reason for this delay in appreciating the hazard was the fact that asbestos dust inhalation produces little in the way of immediate symptoms. Even under the very severe dust conditions which existed at that time noticeable disability took 5 to 7 years to develop and was often mistaken for tuberculosis which was common in factory workers of the day.

The regulations introduced in 1931 were based on Merewether's and Price's study which was mainly concerned with the asbestos textile industry. Although the regulations were applied to some processes in the asbestos cement factories there was no general survey of the other processes in asbestos factories or in the user industries so that inevitably there were groups of workers with unrecognized asbestosis. Although many isolated examples of disease were detected the regulations were not extended widely.

The chief benefit of the 1931 regulations was to improve the conditions of work in certain occupations known to be hazardous and to place the men under continuous medical supervision. In addition to this all men certified as suffering from asbestosis were followed to death and investigated post mortem.

By 1949 it was apparent not only that there were cases of asbestosis occurring outside the prescribed occupations but that both these and the men in prescribed occupations were showing a high incidence of primary lung cancer. As the years passed the serious nature of this second hazard became more obvious; by 1960 half the men certified as suffering from asbestosis were developing lung cancer. Some reassurance was derived from a study which showed that where dust control was adequate to prevent most men from developing asbestosis during their lifetime, the hazard of lung cancer was also eliminated. But the number of men from asbestos factories and user industries who were being certified as suffering from asbestosis and who were dying with lung cancer was still rising year by year.

In 1962 the third hazard of asbestos exposure was revealed by the South African studies linking mesothelioma with relatively trivial exposure to crocidolite. These findings were soon confirmed by studies in the British Isles and in New York. What was previously thought to be a rare but invariably fatal tumour is appearing at about one new case per month from each of the major ship-building ports in Britain. About two cases per month are appearing in London but it is as yet too early to be sure what the incidence is in the country as a whole.

The study of this tumour has raised two new problems. Firstly, standards of safety based on dust counts and the incidence of asbestosis and lung cancer may be of no value in detecting the presence of a mesothelioma hazard. The levels and duration of exposure may be trivial or even undetectable by current methods. Secondly, the high incidence of the tumour in South African crocidolite mining areas and the low incidence in Finland and Canada suggested the tumour may be related to blue asbestos only. Although animal experiments have failed to confirm this, the clinical and epidemiological evidence seems to be compatable with the view that only crocidolite causes mesotheliomas.

Chemical and experimental pathology studies of the various kinds of asbestos have failed to reveal the mechanism by which asbestos causes fibrosis or malignant change. There is no obvious reason why crocidolite should produce different effects from the other fibres. It may be that the differences lie in something quite simple like the shape of the fibre. Anthophyllite appears to be the safest of the commercial fibres in that although there is widespread environmental exposure in Finland it only appears to cause pleural plaques. Asbestosis is relatively uncommon and there is no evidence associating lung cancer with anthophyllite exposure specifically (Noro, 1968). Here is a fibre which produces asbestos bodies in the lung very readily and it may be that inhaled material is all immediately inactivated in this way and most of it remains inactive.

Chrysotile fibres are curly which limits the range of particle size retained in the lung. Evidence as to the proportion of fibres remaining in the lung which are not converted into asbestos bodies is lacking but there is some doubt as to whether mesotheliomas ever occur with this material.

Amosite is physically and geologically more closely related to crocidolite than chrysotile but evidence from the mining areas has failed to reveal a significant incidence of mesotheliomas. It is known to cause pulmonary and pleural fibrosis; the hazards of its use compared with chrysotile are not known.

It is unfortunate that the only soundly based data on morbidity and mortality related to actual levels of dust exposure are related to chrysotile. Regulations based on this data are not directly applicable to mixed exposure or to exposure to other dusts. The new regulations seem to give adequate protection to all workers who are at present known to be at risk from chrysotile but they do not include adequate safeguards to ensure the recognition of undetected or new hazards. Although an attempt is made to deal with the special hazard of crocidolite and mesothelioma it is pure guess work as to whether this will be adequate. To ensure that these new regulations are working effectively where there is a known hazard and to ensure that other hazards are revealed as soon as possible, two additions to the regulations are required. All workers known to be at risk should be subjected to periodic clinical, X-ray and physiological examination. All workers who use asbestos whether they are thought to be at risk or not should be registered and the ultimate causes of death should be analysed for evidence of unrecognized risks.

References

Agricola (1546), *De Natura Fossilium.* Trans. and annot. Bundy and Bundy, Geological Soc. of America Special Paper No. 63, 1955.

Ashcroft, T. (1968), "Asbestos Bodies in Routine Necropsies on Tyneside: A Pathological and Social Study." *Brit. Med. J.*, **1**, 614.

Avril, J. (1968), "Asbestos Bodies in Autopsy Studies of Urban Populations in France." *Proc. 2nd Int. Cong. on the Biological Effects of Asbestos, Dresden.* In press.

Bachirewa, I. (1968), "Right Heart Failure in Asbestosis." *Proc. 2nd Int. Cong. on the Biological Effects of Asbestos, Dresden.* In press.

Beattie, J. and Knox, J. F. (1961), "Studies on the Mineral Content and Particle Size distribution in the Lungs of Asbestos Textile Workers." In *Inhaled Particles and Vapours*, p. 419. Ed. C. N. Davies. London: Pergamon.

Bell, D. and Elmes, P. C. (1968), "Frequency Distribution of Asbestos Bodies in the Lung." *Proc. 2nd Int. Cong. on the Biological Effects of Asbestos, Dresden.* In press.

Bohlig, H. and Jakob, G. (1956), "Neue Gesichtpunkte uber den Lungenkrebs der Asbestarberter." *Dtsch Med. Wschr.*, **81**, 231.

Bohlig, H. (1964), *Staublungener krankungen und ihre Differential*, p. 282, loc. cit. Stuttgart: Georg Thieme Verlag.

Bohlig, H. (1965), "Radiological Classification of Pulmonary Asbestosis." *Ann. N.Y. Acad. Sci.*, **132**, art. 1, 338.

Botham, S. K. and Holt, P. F. (1968a), "The Mechanism of Formation of Asbestos Bodies." *J. Path. and Bact.*, **96**, 443.

Botham, S. K. and Holt, P. F. (1968b), "The Development of Asbestos Bodies." *Proc. 2nd. Int. Cong. on the Biological Effects of Asbestos, Dresden.* In press.

Buchanan, W. D. (1965), "Asbestos and Primary Intrathoracic Neoplasms." *Ann. N.Y. Acad. Sci.*, **132**, art. 1, 507.

Burilkov, T. and Michailova, L. (1970), "Asbestos Content of the Soil and Endemic Pleural Asbestosis." *Env. Res.*, **3**, 443.

Cartier, P. (1955), "Some Clinical Observations of Asbestosis in Mine and Mill Workers." *A.M.A. Arch. Indust. Hlth.*, **11**, 204.

Davis, J. M. (1964), "The Ultra Structure of Asbestos Bodies from Human Lung.' *Brt. J. Exper. Path.*, **45**, 642.

Davis, J. M. (1968), "Electron-Microscope Studies on the Effects of Asbestos Dust on Lung Macrophages Maintained in Organ Culture." *Proc. 2nd Int. Cong. on the Biological Effects of Asbestos, Dresden.* In press.

Elmes, P. C. and Wade, O. L. (1965), "Relationship Between Exposure to Asbestos and Pleural Malignancy in Belfast." *Ann. N.Y. Acad. Sci.*, **132**, art. 1, 549.

Elmes, P. C. and Simpson, M. (1968), "Retrospection Mortality Studies on Pipe Coverers." *Proc. 2nd Int. Cong. on the Biological Effects of Asbestos, Dresden.* In press.

Elmes, P. C. (1971), "International Classification of Radiographs of Pneumoconiosis." *Brit. J. Indust. Med.*, **28**, 93.

Enterline, P. E. (1965), "Mortality Amongst Asbestos Products Workers in the United States." *Ann. N.Y. Acad. Sci.*, **132**, art. 1, 156.

Enticknap, J. B. and Smither, W. J. (1964), "Peritoneal Tumours in Asbestosis." *Brit. J. Indust. Med.*, **21**, 20.

Gaze, R. (1965), "The Physical and Molecular Structure of Asbestos." *Ann. N.Y. Acad. Sci.*, **132**, art. 1, 23.

Hammond, E. C., Selikoff, I. J. and Churg, J. (1965), "Neoplasms Amongst Asbestos Workers in the United States With Special Reference to Intra-abdominal Neoplasms." *Ann. N.Y. Acad. Sci.*, **132**, art. 1, 519.

Harries, P. G. (1968), "The Prevention of Asbestosis in Naval Dockyards." *Proc. 2nd Int. Cong. on the Biological Effects of Asbestos, Dresden.* In press.

Harrington, J. S. (1962), "Natural Occurrence of Oils containing 3,4-Benz Pyrene and Related Substances in Asbestos." *Nature* (*Lond.*), **193,** 43.

Hills, D. W. (1965), "Economics of Dust Control." *Ann. N.Y. Acad. Sci.*, **132,** art. 1, p. 322.

Holmes, S. and Morgan, A. (1968), "The Use of Radioactive Techniques in Studies of the Composition of Asbestos and its Translocation in Rats Following Intra-pleural and Intratracheal Injection." *Proc. 2nd. Int. Cong. on the Biological Effects of Asbestos, Dresden.* In press.

Holmes, S. (1969), Personal communication.

Holt, P. F., Mills, J. and Young, D. K. (1965), "Experimental Asbestosis with Four Types of Fibres: the Importance of Small Particles." *Ann. N.Y. Acad., Sci.*, **132,** art. 1, p. 87.

Hourihane, D. O'B. and McCaughey, W. T. E. (1966), "Pathological Aspects of Asbestosis." *Post Grad. Med. J.*, **42,** 613.

Kiviluoto, R. (1960), "Pleural Calcification as a Sign of Non-occupational Endemic Anthophyllite Asbestosis." *Acta Radiol.* (*Stockh.*) suppl. 194.

Kiviluoto, R. (1965), "Pleural Plaques and Asbestos: Further Observations on Endemic and Other Non-occupational Asbestosis." *N.Y. Acad. Sci.*, **132,** art. **1,** p. 235.

Klosterkötter, W. (1968), "Experimental Studies on the Significance of Fibre Length in Asbestos-fibrosis and Studies on the Impairment of Fibrosis by Poly-vinyl pyridin-n-oxide." *Proc. 2nd Int. Cong. on the Biological Effects of Asbestos, Dresden.* In press.

Knox, J. F. and Beattie, J. (1964), "Distribution of Mineral Particles and Fibres in the Lung After Exposure to Asbestos Dust." *A.M.A. Arch. Indust. Hyg.*, **10,** 30.

Knox, J. F., Holmes, S., Doll, R. and Hill, I. D. (1968), "Mortality from Lung Cancer and Other Causes Among Workers in an Asbestos Textile Factory." *Brit. J. Indust. Med.*, **25,** 293.

McCaughey, W. T. E. (1958), "Primary Tumours of the Pleura." *J. Path. and Bact.*, **76,** 517.

McIver, F. A. (1968), "Results of Inhalation Exposure of Dogs to Chrysotile Asbestos Dust." *Proc. 2nd Int. Cong. on the Biological Effects of Asbestos, Dresden.* In press.

McVittie, J. C. (1965), "Asbestosis in Britain." *Ann. N.Y. Acad. Med.*, **132,** art. 1, p. 128.

Mancuso, T. and El-Attar, A. A. (1968), "Carcinogenic Risk and Duration of Employment Among Asbestos Workers." *Proc. 2nd Int. Cong. on the Biological Effects of Asbestos, Dresden.* In press.

Merewether, E. R. A. and Price (1930), *Report on the Effects of Asbestos Dust on the Lungs and Dust Suppression in the Asbestos Industry.* London: H.M.S.O.

Merewether, E. R. A. (1949), *Annual Report of the Chief Inspector of Factories for the Year* 1947, p. 79. London: H.M.S.O.

Meurmann, L. (1966), "Asbestos Bodies and Pleural Plaques in a Finnish Series of Autopsy Cases." *Acta Pathologica et Microbiol. Scand.* Suppl. 181.

Murray, M. (1907), *Minutes of Evidences: Departmental Cttee on Industrial Diseases*, p. 127. Cmd. Paper 3496. London: H.M.S.O.

Newhouse, M. L. and Thompson, H. (1965), "Mesothelioma of Pleura and Peri-toneum Following Exposure to Asbestos in the London Area." *Brit. J. Indust. Med.*, **22,** 261.

Newhouse, M. L. and Wagner, J. C. (1969), "Validation of Death Certificates in Asbestos Workers." *Brit. J. Ind. Med.*, **26,** 302–8.

Noro, L. (1968), "Occupational and Non-occupational Asbestosis in Finland." *Am. Indust. Hyg. J.*, **29,** 196.

Owen, W. G. (1964), "Diffuse Mesothelioma and Exposure to Asbestos Dust in the Merseyside Area." *Brit. Med. J.*, **2,** 214.

Pernis, B., Vigliani, E. C. and Selikoff, I. J. (1965), "Rheumatoid Factor in Serum of Individuals Exposed to Asbestos." *Ann. N.Y. Acad. Sci.*, **132,** art. 1, p. 112.

Pliny. *Natural History*. Book XIX. IV, 19–20. (Trans. "Loeb's Classics", p. 433.)

Roach, S. A. (1968), *Hygiene Standards for Chrysotile Asbestos Dust*. Published for the Brit. Occupational Hygiene Soc. Oxford: Pergamon Press.

Schepers, G. W. H. (1965), "Discussion on Pathology of Asbestos." *Ann. N.Y. Acad. Sci.*, **132,** art. 1, p. 388.

Seiler, H. (1928), "Case of Pneumoconiosis; Result of Inhalation of Asbestos Dust." *Brit. Med. J.*, **2,** 982.

Selikoff, I. J. (1965), "The Occurrence of Pleural Calcification Among Asbestos Insulation Workers." *Ann. N.Y. Acad. Sci.*, **132,** art. 1, p. 351.

Selikoff, I. J., Churg, J., Hammond, E. C. and Kaffenburgh, J. (1968), "Retrospective Study of Asbestos Neoplasia in Insulation Workers." *Proc. 2nd Int. Cong. on the Biological Effects of Asbestos, Dresden.* In press.

Smith, K. W. (1965), "Trends in the Health of the Asbestos Worker." *Ann. N.Y. Acad. Sci.*, **132,** art. 1, p. 685.

Smither, W. J. (1965), "Secular Changes in Asbestosis in an Asbestos Factory." *Ann. N.Y. Acad. Sci.*, **132,** art. 1, p. 166.

Speil, S. and Leinweber, J. P. (1968), "Asbestos Minerals in Modern Technology." *Proc. 2nd Int. Cong. on Biological Effects of Asbestos, Dresden.* In press.

Stout, A. P. and Murray, M. R. (1942), "Localized Pleural Mesothelioma: Investigation of its Characteristics and Histogenesis." *Arch. Path.*, **34,** 951.

Suzuki, Y., Churg, J. and Smith, W. (1968), "Behaviour of Alveolar Epithelial Cells on Experimental Asbestosis." *Proc. 2nd Int. Cong. on Biological Effects of Asbestos, Dresden.* In press.

Swinburne, L. M. (1968), "Asbestos Related Tumours." *Proc. 2nd Int. Cong. on Biological Effects of Asbestos, Dresden.* In press.

Thomson, J. G. (1965), "Asbestos and the Urban Dweller." *Ann. N.Y. Acad. Sci.*, **132,** art. 1, p. 196.

Timbrell, V. and Skidmore, J. W. (1968), "The Importance of Fibre Length on Experimental Asbestosis." *Proc. 2nd Int. Cong. on Biological Effects of Asbestos, Dresden.* In press.

Turner-Warwick, M. "Immunological Responses in Patients with Asbestosis." Communicated to Symposium on Tissue Responses to Asbestos, Cardiff 1970. Not yet published.

Wagner, J. C., Sleggs, C. A. and Marchand, P. (1960), "Diffuse Pleural Mesotheliomas and Asbestos Exposure on North Western Cape Province." *Brit. J. Indust. Med.*, **17,** 260.

Wagner, J. C., Munday, D. E. and Harington, J. S. (1962), "Histochemical Demonstration of Hyaluronic Acid in Pleural Mesotheliomas." *J. Path. and Bact.*, **84,** 73.

Wagner, J. C. (1968), "Experimental Tumours in Rats Following Intrapleural Inoculation of Asbestos." *Proc. 2nd Int. Cong. on Biological Effects of Asbestos, Dresden.* In press.

Williams, R. and Hugh-Jones, P. (1960), "Lung Function Changes in Asbestosis." *Thorax*, **15,** 109.

Zolov, C., Burilkov, T. and Babadjov, L. (1968), "Probleme der beruflichen und endemischen Asbestose in Bulgarien." II. *Int. Konf. über die biol. Wirkungendes Asbestos, Dresden*, pp. 22–5, April 1968.

Chapter 7

Silicosis and Coalworkers' Pneumoconiosis

C. B. McKerrow

The word pneumoconiosis stems from the Greek *πνεύμων*, lung, and *κόνις*, dust. Strictly, it applies to all conditions in which the lung is affected by inhaled dusts, but in this chapter we shall consider only two examples—the diseases due to the inhalation of free silica and those arising from breathing coal dust. It is only in the last quarter century that coalworkers' pneumoconiosis has been clearly recognized as having a different aetiology from silicosis. Indeed until 1943, the Workmen's Compensation Acts recognized for compensation only men whose radiographs showed a characteristic silicotic appearance. It will be convenient to consider the aetiology, incidence and pathology of the two conditions separately while discussing clinical features and treatment together.

Silicosis

Occurrence

Silicosis results from the inhalation of particles of silicon dioxide (SiO_2), often referred to as "free" or "uncombined" silica to differentiate it from the various silicates. Free silica dusts are produced from a great number of industrial sources, as suggested by Table 1 which gives the numbers of workers newly certified as having industrial pulmonary disease in those industries in which silicosis is a hazard.

Sandstone contains between 75 and 95% free silica and those at risk include not only men who fabricate sandstone blocks for building, but also the numerous masons working in builders' or sculptors' yards. In the past the use of sandstone for grinding was an important source of silicosis, but this has been virtually eliminated by the use of artificial abrasive wheels.

Granite has a crystalline structure and contains feldspar, quartz and mica, the percentage of free silica being rather less than sandstone. It is a good building stone on account of its toughness and excellent wearing properties and these qualities make it valuable also for road making, kerbstones and as a constituent of concrete.

Thirty new cases of pneumoconiosis were certified in 1969 among slate miners and splitters. The majority of these will be of silicosis as slate contains about 40% quartz.

The pottery industry has been a source of silicosis since 1720 when John Astbury introduced calcined flint into his chinaware. Today the remaining silicosis hazard in the industry is still from flint; in earthenware it is used as an ingredient of the liquid slip from which the article is made. The danger arises initially in milling the flint and then either from spillage of the slip which will dry and can then be brushed off as a powder, or from fettling the article before it is fired. Also protective clothing made of cotton can harbour particles which, after drying, can be released into the breathing zone of the worker. Chinaware does not contain flint, but until 1947 powdered flint was used to bed the china biscuit before firing and constituted the main source of silicosis in the industry. In 1947 this use of flint was prohibited and calcined alumina substituted, and today powdered bedding materials are being dispensed with entirely. Table 1 shows that the numbers of pottery workers compensated fell between 1957 and 1969 from 233 new cases to 31.

Table 1

First diagnosis of compensatable disease in industries with a silica risk, excluding coal mining
(From the annual reports of the Ministry of Pensions and National Insurance and the Ministry of Social Security and the Department of Health and Social Security)

Industry	1957	1969
Foundry workers	259	40
Furnace dismantling	13	2
Pottery	233	31
Quarrying	6	10
Refractories	51	16
Sandblasting	9	1
Sandstone	41	8
Slate mining	13	21
Slate splitting	14	16
Steel dressers	77	14
Tunnellers	5	3

Foundry work may involve the risk of silicosis at a number of points in the process. Firstly, moulding sands are mixtures containing silica and sand with a binder such as ball clay, china clay, etc. The moulder is unlikely to be exposed to high dust concentrations when the moulding material is wet, but fettling is relatively dusty. A risk of silicosis also arises in dismantling furnaces lined with silica brick. Again, there has been a large decline in new cases certified in the twelve-year period.

Silicosis can result from any quarrying, tunnelling or mining operation in which quartz dust is present. It is occasionally found in coal-miners as certain jobs underground expose them predominantly to stone dust; these include ripping to increase the height of an underground roadway, or hard heading in which a tunnel or "drift" is made through the rock.

In addition silicosis may occur in many occupations such as the manufacture of refractory products and abrasive soaps, in flint crushing, handling diatomaceous earth, etc., but the recognition of the risk in these occupations has usually reduced the problem to small proportions.

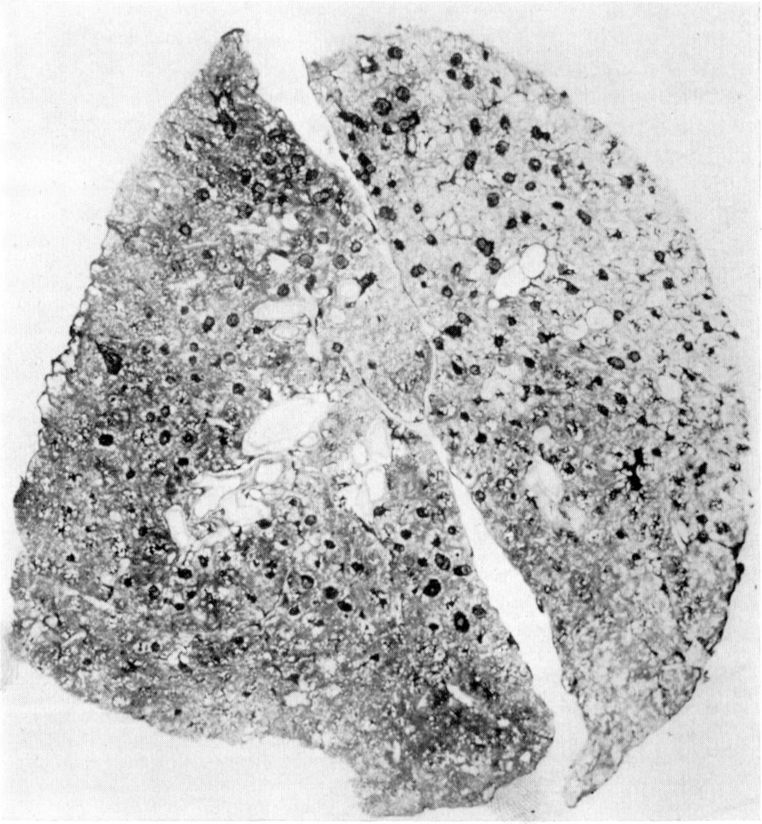

FIG. 1. Whole lung section showing widespread silicotic nodules.

Pathology

The essential feature of the pathology of silicosis is fibrosis, usually commencing as hard nodules about 1 mm in diameter but increasing in size and coalescing as the disease progresses (Fig. 1).

Microscopically these silicotic nodules are seen to originate in the peri-bronchial lymphoid tissue in association with particles of silica taken up by large macrophages. Once in the lymphoid tissue the macrophages become surrounded by fibroblasts giving place later to collagenous fibres. A continuous sequence of new fibroblasts, later to be turned into collagen, is laid down at the periphery of the nodule and this sequence gives the typical whorled appearance of the silicotic nodule. With the passage of time neighbouring nodules coalesce (Fig. 2).

Tuberculous infection is potentiated by silica and may arise either independently in the lung or, more usually, cause modification of the silicotic process, so-called silico-tuberculosis. The resulting lesion is a densely fibrotic nodule. It is often irregular in shape and histologically

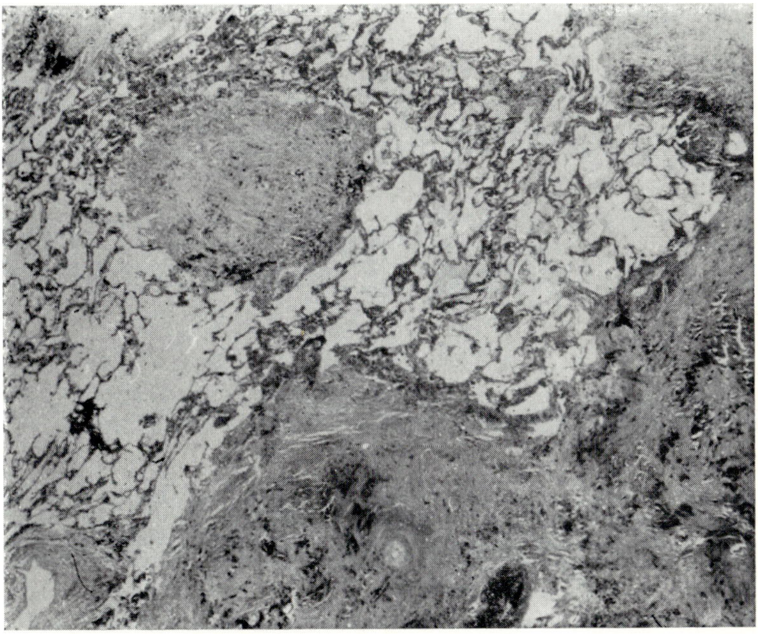

FIG. 2. Histological section showing single and confluent silicotic nodules.

both caseation and small areas of calcification are common. Tubercle bacilli and giant cells are usually scanty and may be absent, and it can be impossible to prove a tuberculous aetiology. When present in coalminers the lesion is pigmented by the associated coal dust.

Cases of acute silicosis are still seen in tunnellers exposed to enormous concentrations of rock dust, and also among those in highly siliceous dust mixed with an alkali, as in the manufacture of abrasive soap powders. It has been suggested that the activity of the silica is potentiated by being rendered more soluble in an alkaline solution, but there is little direct evidence. Microscopically the lesions show a diffuse fibrotic picture with early silicotic islands.

Theories of Aetiology

Many theories have been advanced to explain the development of the silicotic nodule. An early idea that the sharp quartz particles damaged the lung tissue has been discredited by showing in animal experiments that harder materials such as carborundum or diamond cause no similar damage.

Gye and Kettle (1922) suggested that the toxic action of silica results from the liberation of silicic acid which acts as a cell poison. Several facts supported this hypothesis: for instance, the liberation of silicic acid could be inhibited by coating the particle with the hydroxides of iron or aluminium, and this also rendered it non-toxic. But there were discrepancies in the relationship between the amount of silicic acid released in animal experiments and the amount of fibrosis produced (King *et al.*, 1956). Also silica within a semipermiable membrane did not cause silicosis even though the liberation of silicic acid was unimpeded.

These difficulties forced attention on the relative toxicity of mono- and polysilicic acids. Polysilicic acids have potent damaging effects when injected into small animals, by increasing capillary permeability, and by inhibition of various cell enzyme systems. It has also been postulated that one action of phagocytes containing quartz may be the formation of a collagen precursor which in turn collects monosilicic acid from the quartz surface and stores it until it polymerizes and changes procollagen to collagen (Holt, 1957).

Marks *et al.* (1956) showed that in vitro the toxic effects of various dusts on monocytes related to their fibrogenic activity, suggesting that injury to the phagocytic cell by dust is the stimulus for fibrous tissue formation. Harington and Allison (1965) studied the nature of this primary damage to the phagocytic cell claiming that when silica dust enters it, hydrolytic enzymes contained in their lysosomes are released. These enzymes instead of remaining in the phagosomes of the cells as in bacterial phagocytosis are discharged into the cell cytoplasm itself and lead to its death.

A still more recent theory suggests that the destruction of the phagocyte is due to electron transfer between the phagocytic cell membrane and special sites, "electron traps", in the silica substance (Robock, 1967). The toxic effect can be attributed to a surface characteristic of silica leading to catalytic changes in organic molecules adsorbed onto it.

There is evidence that protein adsorbed on quartz acts as an antigen and Vigliani and Pernis (1958) reviewed the concept that the hyaline material in silicotic lesions might be the result of an antigen-antibody reaction. The main points of evidence leading to this theory were first the large amounts of gamma globulins present in the hyaline tissue of silicosis, secondly the augmentation of activity in the reticulo-endothelial system and variations in nonspecific immunity after the introduction of free silica dust, and lastly the appearance of anti-polysaccharide antibodies in the serum of some silicotic patients. It was claimed that silica dust causes macrophages to set free substances, probably polysaccharides, which are auto-antigenic. An attraction of the hypothesis is that it could explain the increase in pathogenic activity of quartz dust following tuberculous infection because mycobacteria have been shown to cause nonspecific stimulation of the reticulo-endothelial system.

The final answer remains to be proved. A useful review of the earlier theories is given by Nagelschmidt (1960). It seems unlikely today that the silica solubility theories are tenable; the attractive work of Allison and Harington gives a good explanation of the destruction of the macrophage and some form of auto-immunological action could account for the subsequent development of the silicotic nodule; but it must be admitted that almost all the experimental evidence relates to laboratory animals, often with injected rather than inhaled dusts, and its relevance to human silicosis is uncertain.

Coalworkers' Pneumoconiosis

Occurrence

Lung disease in coal-miners has been a known hazard of the industry at least since the mid-seventeenth century, and was then attributed to some "virulent vapour" arising from the coal. It is now accepted that the respirable portion of the dust itself is the only aetiological agent and that its effect varies in relation to its concentration and composition. Following the introduction of size-selective dust sampling instruments in British coal mines it has been possible to measure the mass concentration of airborne particles in the respirable size range at the coal face on a large scale. Correlation of the measurements with changes observed in X-ray films of the mining population have shown that the mass concentration of the respirable dust is the dominant aetiological factor (Jacobsen *et al.*, 1971).

The amount of airborne dust (Fig. 3) depends on the activity of men and machines at the coal face and on the efficiency of the local air ventilation. The concentration of respirable airborne particles varies widely from place to place and from minute to minute, reaching high peaks after activities such as shot firing, but an average figure of 5 or 6 mg/m^3 might be representative of the industry as a whole in this country.

The composition of coal dust likewise varies greatly from one mine to another especially in relation to the job being undertaken. Representative values of airborne respirable dust might be 60% coal, 35% mineral matter such as kaolin, and 4% free silica. The silica comes largely from the rock of floor and roof and its concentration can be much higher in certain occupations (see "Silicosis" above).

The "rank" of coal is a complex index. Coal represents the remains of vast swamp forests covering the land some 250 million years ago. As the dead vegetation sank into the bog it began the gradual change which converted it into peat, brown coal, bituminous coal, and eventually into anthracite. The early stages of the series are called low rank coals

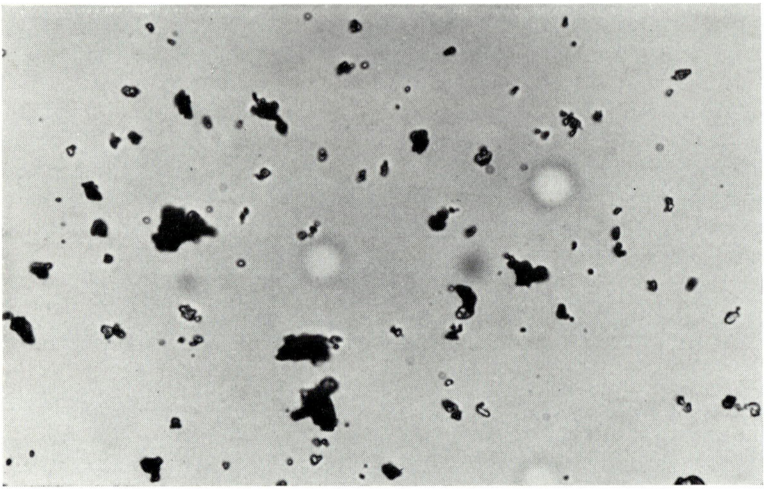

FIG. 3. Airborne coal-dust particles. (Scale 1 mm = 1 μ.)

and the final stages high rank. The change is produced by bacteria and fungi at the peat stage and by high temperatures in oxygen-free conditions at the final stage. Chemically the series is characterized by a gradual reduction in the content of volatile matter and of moisture and by an associated increase in the carbon content and in its hardness. The concept linking "rank" of coal with incidence of pneumoconiosis arose from the high prevalence of the disease in the South Wales anthracite areas with high rank coal. The harmful effects previously attributed to rank can now be more easily explained in terms of the high mass concentration of respirable dust in these particular mines.

The hard, high-rank anthracite seams of South Wales are associated with a coarse dust usually having a low mineral content, although there is conflicting evidence on the relation between the rank of coal and the size distribution of particles within the respirable range. The association between rank of coal and the mineral or ash content of the airborne dust depends on the structure of the seams and may be influenced more by different mining methods than by any fundamental geological properties.

One of the major difficulties in attempting to correlate the various factors such as dust concentration and composition in a mine with the incidence of pneumoconiosis is that the mine environment has changed greatly over the years. Improved ventilation underground may have reduced the average dust concentration in the pits by a factor of one half to one third in the last twenty years. But the large increase in mechanical means of winning coal has made further reduction difficult as mechanization is always associated with higher fine dust production, and since 1955 the percentage of output by mechanical means has risen from about 10% to over 90%.

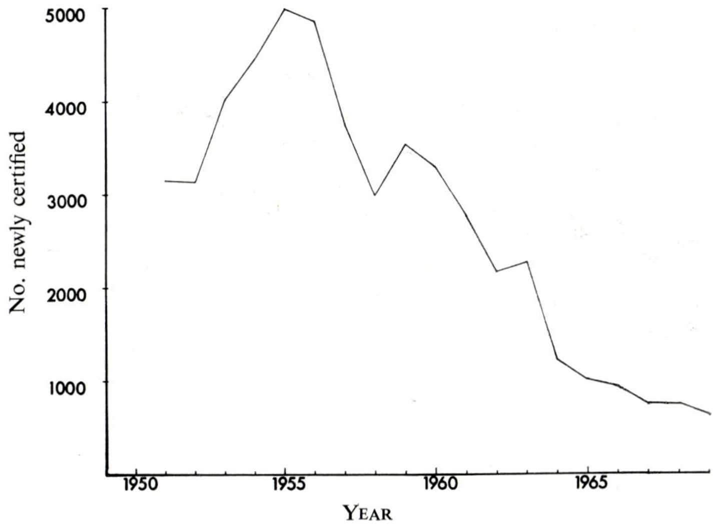

FIG. 4. Miners newly certified for compensation for pneumoconiosis in the United Kingdom.
(Sources: Ministry of Power Digests of Pneumoconoisis Statistics H.M.S.O. Annual Reports of the Ministry of Social Security, and Department of Health and Social Security.)

Figure 4 shows the numbers of coal-miners newly certified each year as having compensatable pneumoconiosis. The initial rise in certifications is mainly due to relaxation of the criteria for certification in the National Insurance (Industrial Injuries) Act of 1948. Although contraction of the industry may have slightly reduced the applications in recent years, the trend is large enough to indicate a real improvement in working conditions.

Pathology

Pneumoconiosis of coalworkers is divisible into simple pneumoconiosis—having little harmful effect on the lung—and complicated pneumoconiosis or progressive massive fibrosis (PMF) arising on the simple disease and leading to gross pulmonary impairment both in structure and function.

Simple pneumoconiosis. The lesion of simple pneumoconiosis (Fig. 5) is less fibrotic than that of simple silicosis. Coal dust collects in foci up to 5 mm in diameter around the small bronchioles after having been transported from the alveoli by phagocytes. A small amount of reticulin fibres develop at these sites and some may proceed to collagen, but this

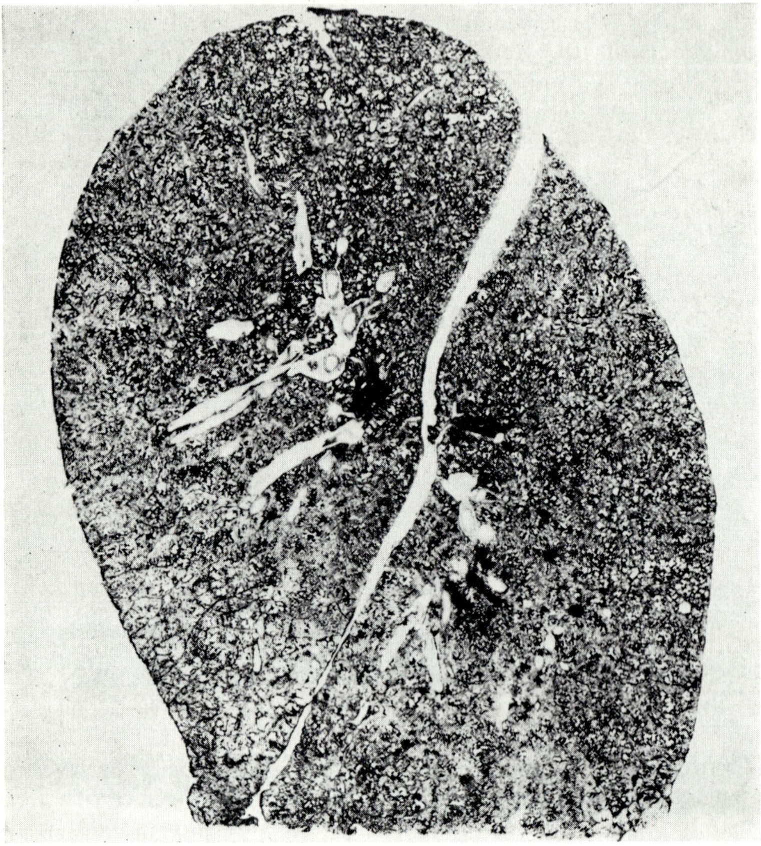

FIG. 5. Simple pneumoconiosis. A whole lung section of a miner who died aged 58 after 44 years' work underground. It shows numerous small dust foci associated with focal emphysema.

is considerably less than is found in silicosis. Around the coal foci the air spaces become dilated, a condition described by Gough (1947) as focal emphysema. The mechanism of the production of these emphysematous spaces is not clear, but most pathologists favour a mechanical explanation in which the dust foci interfere in some way with the function of the respiratory bronchioles. The focal emphysema of simple pneumoconiosis must be clearly differentiated from panacinar

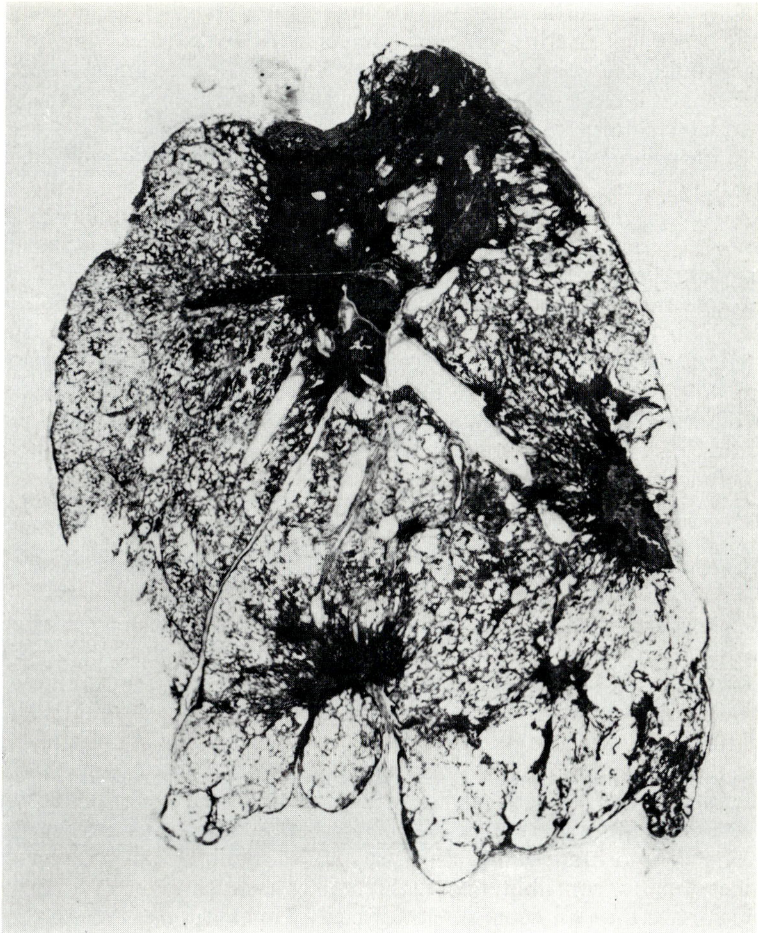

FIG. 6. Complicated pneumoconiosis. A whole lung section of a miner who died aged 62 after 33 years' work underground. There is extensive progressive massive fibrosis in the upper lobe and severe emphysema especially at the base.

emphysema in which the condition is generalized and results in mechanical impairment of ventilation. Simple pneumoconiosis is a condition entirely produced by the dust inhaled; it will not increase in severity in the absence of further dust inhalation, nor will it regress.

Complicated pneumoconiosis. In complicated pneumoconiosis the dust collections become embedded in dense areas of fibrous tissue (Fig. 6). The massive fibrosis tends to occur in the upper parts of the lung and is usually bilateral. The centres of the masses are very ischaemic due to obliterative endarteritis and may be replaced by cavities containing black fluid, the source of the clinical condition called melanoptysis. The masses are distinguishable from those of silicosis by the absence of a nodular pattern.

In the production of these lesions there is considerable contraction of the lung tissue, and this often causes basal emphysema and bullae surrounding the masses themselves. Thus lung function is impaired far beyond the actual areas of complicated pneumoconiosis. The ischaemic changes reduce the pulmonary vascular bed leading to pulmonary hypertension, right ventricular hypertrophy and congestive heart failure.

Caplan (1953) drew attention to a modified form of complicated pneumoconiosis in miners with rheumatoid arthritis. The lesions in Caplan's syndrome are numerous and discrete, often of only 1 to 2 cms in diameter (Fig. 7). They have similar distribution to the ordinary lesions of complicated pneumoconiosis and histologically the main differences are a greater tendency for calcification at the centres and an active inflammatory zone at the periphery.

Theories of Aetiology

Simple pneumoconiosis. It is generally accepted that the extent of simple pneumoconiosis is related to the quantity and composition of dust retained in the lung. For instance, Rivers *et al.* (1960) demonstrated a good relationship between total weight of dust in lungs examined after death and the radiological category of simple pneumoconiosis in life. But the radiograph is not a sensitive indicator of small amounts of dust retention as the lungs of miners without radiological abnormality may contain ten times the weight of dust than those of a town dweller.

The composition of the dust may affect radiological appearance, mineral matter contributing over three times as much to the radiological appearance than an equal weight of coal (Rossiter *et al.*, 1966).

Complicated pneumoconiosis. Why do some men with simple pneumoconiosis develop the complicated disease? The answer is still not known with certainty and three hypotheses have had support at various times.

The silica theory suggested that the silica content of the dust causes progressive massive fibrosis and that without it only simple pneumoconiosis can develop. However, there is not a sufficiently good relationship between incidence of complicated pneumoconiosis and quartz content of respirable dust, although lungs with complicated pneumoconiosis do contain significantly more quartz than those without. Animal experiments indicate that at least 10% of quartz would be needed in respired air to produce fibrosis, and this hypothesis has been generally abandoned.

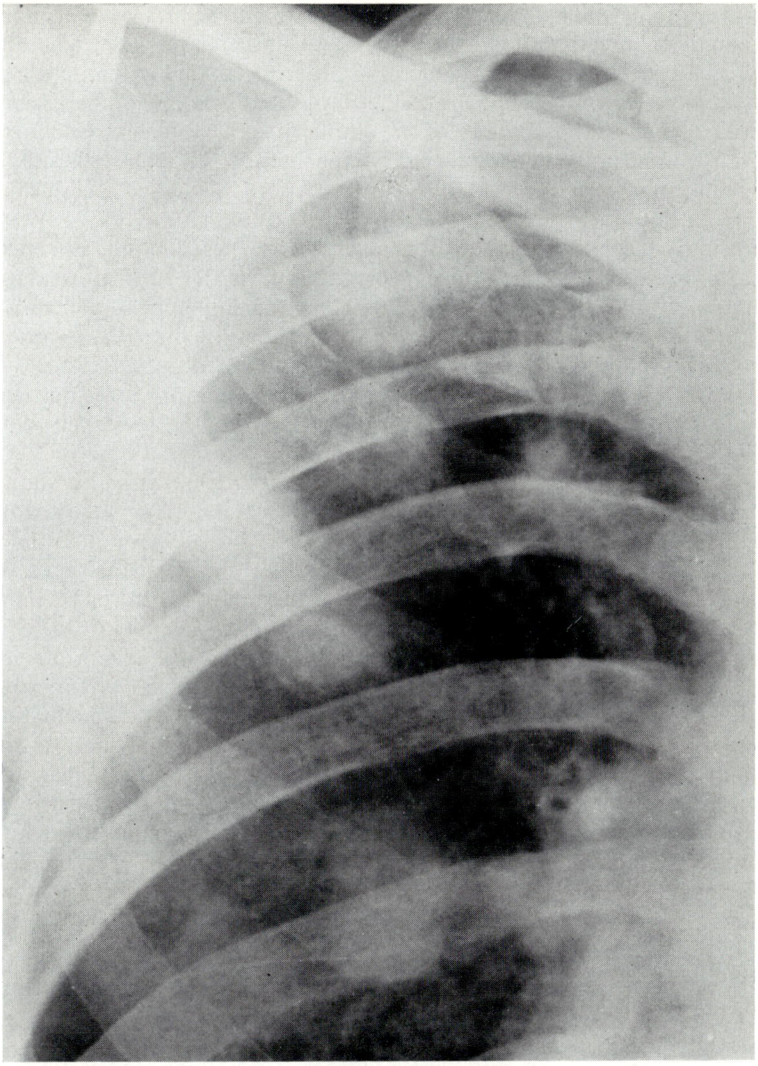

FIG. 7. X-ray of right upper lobe showing lesions of Caplan's syndrome in a coal-miner.

A quarter of a century ago it was demonstrated that in 40% of autopsies of miners with complicated pneumoconiosis, tubercle bacilli could be recovered from the lungs, and the general similarity of the pathology to fibroid tuberculosis suggested a possible common aetiology. Research has failed to substantiate the hypothesis. Mantoux positivity is not higher in complicated than simple pneumoconiosis nor has the attack rate of PMF fallen in relation to falls in the risk of exogenous tuberculous infection. Lastly, short-term anti-tuberculous chemotherapy has not been proved to influence the progression rate of complicated pneumoconiosis. The attack rate of complicated pneumoconiosis seems better related to the category of the simple pneumoconiosis: Cochrane (1962) found an attack rate of 0·7% per annum in men with simple pneumoconiosis category 1, 2·6% with category 2, and 4·2% with category 3. Recent results from serial X-ray examinations of working miners by the National Coal Board agree with these findings but show that in the whole country the expected attack rate of PMF in working miners is rather lower in those with Category 3 simple pneumoconiosis (McLintock *et al.*, 1971). But Cochrane's studies included ex-miners as well as working miners and this may have accounted for some, at least, of the difference. In the coal fields of Great Britain as a whole, this new study has shown an attack rate of PMF in coal-face workers with ILO Category 2 or more simple pneumoconiosis to be 1·5% per year, but there is considerable variation in different areas. It has also shown that progression of simple pneumoconiosis as well as its initial category increases the liability to develop PMF.

Although Caplan established the syndrome bearing his name on an association between miners with a well-defined radiological picture and rheumatoid arthritis, recent work (Wagner and McCormick, 1967) has demonstrated the presence of rheumatoid factor in the serum of men with complicated pneumoconiosis not typical of Caplan's syndrome, and more often free of overt rheumatoid arthritis. However, rheumatoid factor was not present in all men with complicated pneumoconiosis and immunohistological methods were used to demonstrate a particular histological type of lung lesion associated with a high incidence of positive rheumatoid factor tests. These lungs were found to include Caplan's syndrome as expected, but also lungs with PMF showing vasculitis with plasma cell infiltration. Thus it seems likely that an immunological mechanism plays a part in producing some, but probably not all, lesions of complicated pneumoconiosis.

Diagnosis and Assessment

Simple pneumoconiosis and simple silicosis. The simple forms both of coalworkers' pneumoconiosis and of silicosis may be symptomless, especially in the young. Severe dyspnoea is usually due to chronic bronchitis or the coincident presence of panacinar emphysema. Diagnosis must therefore be radiological supported by history of exposure to the dust. The length of exposure varies widely: acute silicosis has been reported following exposures of less than a year, but in coalworkers radiological changes in under five years are unusual.

The radiological appearances consist of discrete round or irregular shadows of any size from 0·5 mm to 10 mm, but characteristically those of silicosis are larger than are found in the coalworker.

The assessment of extent of the pneumoconioses must be based on a quantitative interpretation of chest radiographs and a classification has been prepared by the International Labour Office (1958), but is at present under revision.

The ILO Classification (1958). The outline of the classification is shown in Table 2 giving the three main parameters, the type of opacity, its

Table 2

The form of the International Labour Office radiographic classification (1958)

	No. pneumo-coniosis	*Suspect*	*Pneumoconiosis*			
Type of opacity			Small opacities			Large opacities
Qualitative features	0	Z	p	m	n	A B C
Quantitative features			1 2 3	1 2 3	1 2 3	

qualitative feature and its profusion. The opacities may be linear, small or large. Their quality is defined by "p", "m" or "n" (or "p", "q", "r") if small and predominantly round (Table 3).

Each of the qualitative categories of small opacities may be quantitated by the figures 1, 2, 3 and extent of the large opacities by the letters "A", "B" and "C" indicating the proportion of lung fields obscured by opacities. It should be noted that the denominator in the fraction is *one* lung field, even if the PMF is bilateral. Examples of the classifications are given in Figs. 8–10.

The value of any classification depends on its reproducibility, not only when used by one observer but also between them. The International Labour Office has prepared sets of Standard radiographs for comparison with unknown films. Using these, experienced observers can place between 80 and 90% of films of simple pneumoconiosis in the same category on two occasions when about 20% of films being read are abnormal. Various techniques can be employed in classifying films. If they are examined by more than one observer an agreed interpretation could be obtained by discussion. There are several disadvantages of this, not the least being that the agreed reading may depend as much on the personality of the observer as on his skill! But more important, the agreed reading may discard information by ignoring the fact that radiological abnormality is continuous and not a

Table 3

Definitions of the ILO Classification (1958)

Qualitative		*No pneumoconiosis*
	O	No radiographic evidence of pneumoconiosis.
		Suspect opacities
	Z	Increased lung markings.
		Simple pneumoconiosis
	p	Punctiform opacities. Size up to 1·5 mm.
	m	Micro-nodular or miliary opacities. Greatest diameter between 1·5 and 3 mm.
	n	Nodular opacities. Size between 3 and 10 mm.
Quantitative	Category 1	A small number of opacities in an area equivalent to at least two anterior rib spaces and at the most not greater than one-third of the two lung fields.
	Category 2	Opacities more numerous and diffuse than in category 1 and distributed over most of the lung fields.
	Category 3	Very numerous profuse opacities covering the whole or nearly the whole of the lung fields.
		Complicated pneumoconiosis
	A	An opacity having a longest diameter of between 1 and 5 cm, or several opacities each greater than 1 cm, the sum of whose longest diameters does not exceed 5 cm.
	B	One or more opacities, larger or more numerous than those in category A, whose combined area does not exceed one-third of one lung field.
	C	One or more large opacities, whose combined area exceeds one-third of one lung field.

discrete process. This concept has been developed by Wise and Oldham (1963) and by Liddell (1963) who has made it the basis of an extended classification (Liddell and May, 1966) by dividing the spectrum from normality to extreme abnormality into a twelve-point rather than a four-point scale. In this the basic four categories remain, but the observer is allowed to record whether, during the process of classification, a neighbouring category was considered as a serious alternative. If so, this category is recorded after the main one. Thus, category 2/1 is a film of category 2, but category 1 was also seriously considered.

The UICC/Cincinnati classification. This new classification is based on that of the present ILO 1958 scheme and has been developed by the International Union Against Cancer (UICC) for use in the pneumoconioses including asbestosis (1970). It employs the twelve-point

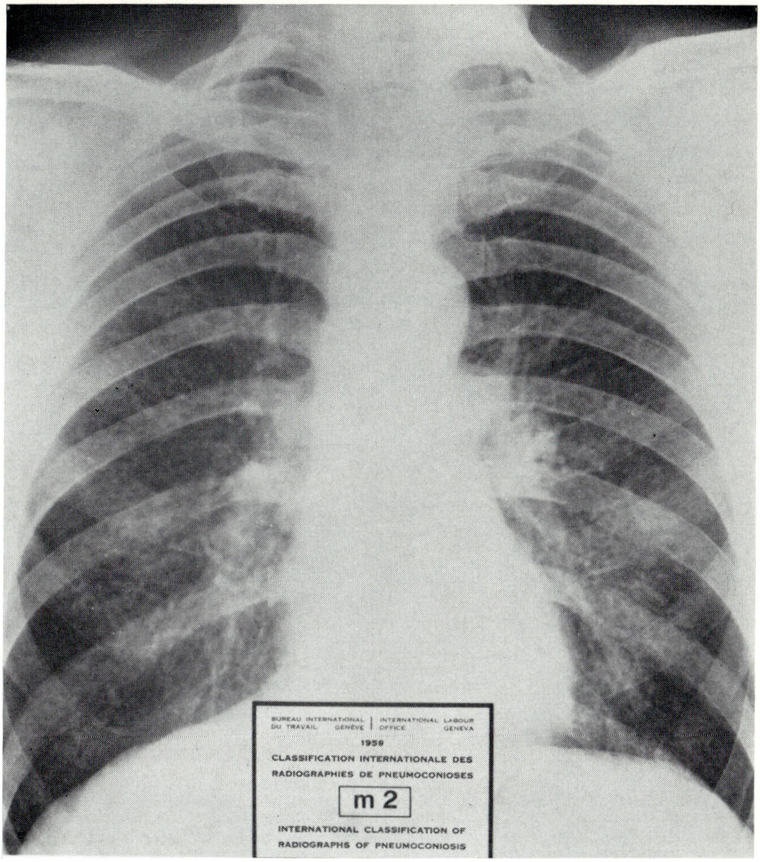

FIG. 8. ILO Standard Radiograph of simple pneumoconiosis category 2 with "m" opacities.

scale discussed above and, in addition, small opacities are sub-divided into rounded (as in the present ILO Scheme) and "irregular". This new irregular group has four categories, 0–3 and is relevant to the small irregular appearances seen in asbestosis and other pneumoconioses. Pleural thickening for which a single symbol was used in the ILO 1958 Scheme, is included in the main classification and divided into "calcified" and "non-calcified". Also ill-defined cardiac outline and diaphragmatic outline are separately classified. The new classification has been designed to extend the present ILO one and thus the levels of grading of rounded opacities (simple coalworkers' pneumoconiosis) are similar in the old and new classifications if the second figure of the twelve-point scale is disregarded, e.g. a category 2 film in the ILO 1958

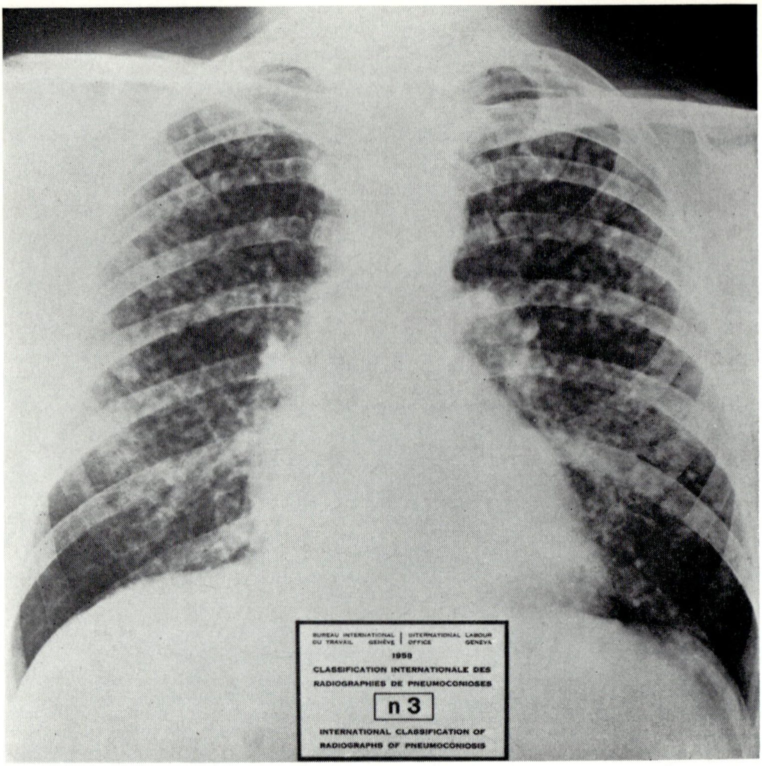

FIG. 9. ILO Standard Radiograph of simple pneumoconiosis category 3 with "n" opacities.

Classification will be a category 2/1, 2/2 or 2/3 in the UICC/Cincinnati Scheme.

Differential diagnosis. There are many non-industrial conditions giving nodular lesions in the chest radiograph, and in addition it is not uncommon for a man to have had exposure to several mineral dusts in his working life.

Of the non-industrial causes of confusion, sarcoidosis, mitral stenosis, haemosiderosis, metastases, and possibly various virus, bacterial and fungoid infections may mimic simple pneumoconiosis and silicosis. Miliary tuberculosis is now rare. In sarcoidosis the mediastinal lymph nodes are commonly enlarged, and constitutional disturbance and the short history in relation to total dust exposure may also help. In mitral stenosis and haemosiderosis the dense and small nodules may be impossible to distinguish from silicosis, but the contour of the heart may be a help in mitral stenosis. The general condition of the subject should

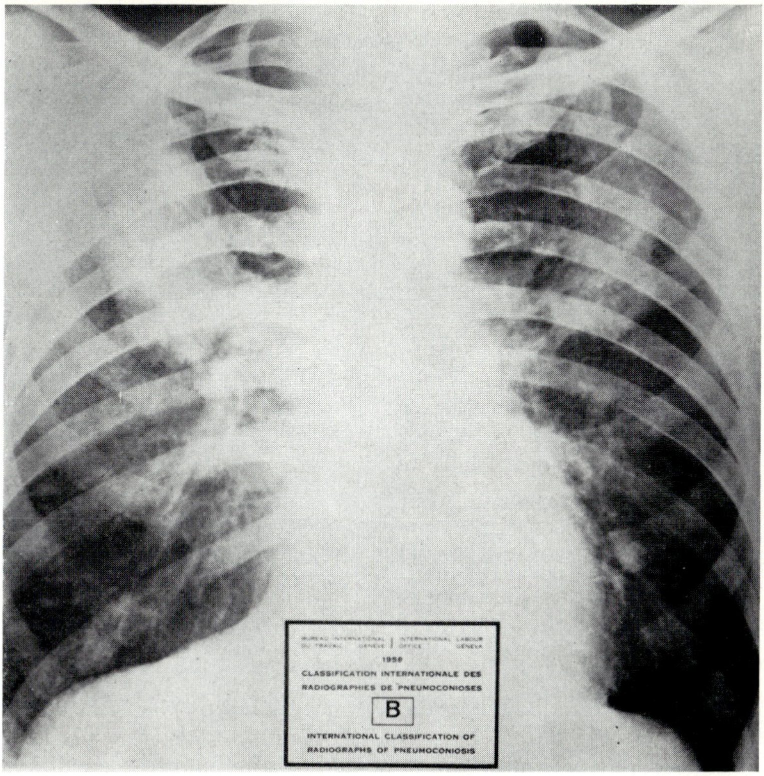

FIG. 10. ILO Standard Radiograph showing complicated pneumoconiosis category B.

serve to differentiate miliary carcinomatosis in the lung. Occasionally carcinoma of the thyroid produces haematogenous secondary deposits in the lung while the general condition of the patient remains surprisingly good. Bacterial and viral infections causing X-ray changes should not cause confusion with pneumoconiosis although occasionally serial X-ray films are necessary.

It is always advisable to take note of any other occupational exposure that a man may have had at any time in his life. Particularly asbestosis may be missed and occasionally beryllium disease can follow a period of exposure sufficiently short not to be spontaneously mentioned. Two other occupational exposures sometimes overlooked arise from farming small holdings and pigeon keeping.

Complicated Pneumoconiosis and Silico-Tuberculosis

Breathlessness on exertion is the characteristic symptom of both conditions. Typically it will vary little from time to time and its severity relates to the area of lung destruction and to age. The extent of dyspnoea can be assessed by the defined questions (Medical Research Council, 1960) of the Medical Research Council's bronchitis questionnaire dividing breathlessness into grades (Table 4) ranging from no abnormal

Table 4

Dyspnoea grades
(Medical Research Council bronchitis questionnaire, 1966.)

	Question	*Reply*	*Grade of dyspnoea*
14a	Are you troubled by shortness of breath when hurrying on level ground or walking up a slight hill?	Neg 14a	Grade 1
		Pos 14a Neg 14b and c	Grade 2
14b	Do you get short of breath walking with other people of your own age on level ground?	Pos 14a and b Neg 14c	Grade 3
14c	Do you have to stop for breath when walking at your own pace on level ground?	Pos 14a, b, c	Grade 4

breathlessness (Grade 1) to severe dyspnoea (Grade 4). Wheeze is usual especially on expiration, but, as with breathlessness, it tends to be constant from day to day. Symptoms are often modified by additional bronchitis.

Bignall (1969) found that some 30% of a random sample of miners complained of chest pain compared with about 7% of non-miners. Pain or discomfort was in general substernal or in the left chest and arm, and appeared to be related to exertion. However, there was no evidence of excessive ECG abnormality in the group nor was the incidence of chest pain related to the amount of pneumoconiosis. Perhaps these miners had an increased awareness of chest discomfort. In addition to these angina-like pains, transient sharp pains resembling those of pleurisy, are not uncommon in men with complicated pneumoconiosis. They tend to flit from one area to another and pleural effusion is uncommon.

Progressive massive fibrosis and silico-tuberculosis show irregular shadows on the radiographs of at least one cm diameter and often involving more than half of the total lung field, and its classification has already been discussed.

Occasionally miners with advanced complicated pneumoconiosis may expectorate large volumes of black sputum from cavities within the massive lesions. This melanoptysis is often associated with a bronchitic attack, but there is little other constitutional disturbance. The condition must be differentiated from tuberculous cavitation in the miner in which there is considerable constitutional effect and the prognosis is poor.

Differential diagnosis. Differential diagnosis of silico-tuberculosis and complicated pneumoconiosis lies between fibroid tuberculosis and carcinoma of the lung. It is impossible to eliminate the possibility that a small apical opacity may be tuberculous, but in the coalworker the presence of simple pneumoconiosis of Category 2 or above and the absence of constitutional symptoms and signs favour complicated pneumoconiosis. Tubercle bacilli are now found in less than 2% of men with complicated pneumoconiosis, in the United Kingdom, and infection by anonymous (opportunist) mycobacteria is about as common.

Carcinoma of the lung may resemble unilateral "A" shadows of complicated pneumoconiosis, but with the following points of difference: the PMF shadow is typically of irregular outline, often with an ill-defined edge when small; it is usually apical initially. Category B shadows of complicated pneumoconiosis are seldom unilateral. Even when a PMF shadow is close to the hilum there is usually a relatively clear area intervening. The frequency of death from lung carcinoma is lower in workers in the coal-mining industry than in other occupational groups of comparable age. Goldman showed that the survival rates of men with lung cancer was improved in presence of pneumoconiosis (Goldman, 1965), and Ashley (1967) has suggested that the mechanism may have an immunologic component, tending to enhance the lung's defences against tumour cells. Thus a high category of simple pneumoconiosis would tend to favour a diagnosis of PMF and make one of carcinoma less likely.

Bronchitis

Bronchitis needs special mention in relation to dust diseases of the lung in view of the possibility that it is caused by industrial dusts, and also because of the disability it produces in many cases of industrial lung disease.

Its prevalence is high among miners especially in the Welsh coalfields; the Registrar General's Decennial Supplement (1951) gives a standardized mortality ratio for bronchitis in the age group 20 to 64 years of 135 for all miners and of 200 for face-workers. But the bronchitic death rate is high in all heavy industry. Similarly, rates of incapacity for bronchitis are high in all heavy occupations other than agriculture. Some at least of this morbidity can be attributed to general air pollution from the towns in which heavy industry is situated and still more from smoking. The relation of chronic bronchitis to occupation is discussed in a Medical Research Council report (1966) which emphasizes the difficulty of ascribing an occupational origin to bronchitis in the individual, particularly as there are no features distinguishing bronchitis in industry from that outside. Some preliminary results from research by the National Coal Board suggest a statistically significant level of association between the amount of inhaled dust and the prevalence of symptoms of cough and phlegm in men under 45 years, but again emphasises the important effect of smoking at all ages (Rae *et al.*, 1971).

Lung Function

Simple pneumoconiosis and silicosis. Most surveys of lung function in simple pneumoconiosis and silicosis have shown ventilatory capacity to be slightly lower than expected, but with little or no relation to the radiological category. Unless chronic bronchitis is present, these small changes are unlikely to be accompanied by respiratory disability.

Some widening of the alveolar-arterial tension difference for oxygen with a slight reduction in the transfer factor for the lung has been noted in simple pneumoconiosis and is probably due to some unevenness of ventilation and perfusion (Brasseur, 1963). Englert and De Coster (1965) and others suggested that these cases were associated especially with simple pneumoconiosis of the pinhead type, and the observation was confirmed by Lyons *et al.* (1967) who found a gas transfer defect in the lungs in ten of sixteen miners with pinhead type simple pneumoconiosis but in none of eleven men whose opacities were of the micronodular type. It may be that there is a small group of men with simple pneumoconiosis whose lung function differs qualitatively from the rest. In advanced simple pneumoconiosis lung compliance tends to be slightly reduced in men below 40 years and a similar change is seen in silicosis and silico-tuberculosis.

Complicated pneumoconiosis and silico-tuberculosis. Either disease when advanced may cause severe impairment of lung function by occupying space within the thorax and by distorting the remaining lung tissue, often causing large areas of compensatory emphysema especially at the bases. These changes lead to impairment of ventilatory ability especially in older men. The massive lesions are mainly avascular and cause reduction in the pulmonary vascular bed leading ultimately to congestive cardiac failure.

Cochrane *et al.* (1961) have shown that the decline in ventilatory capacity determined by the $FEV_{1 \cdot 0}$ relates approximately to the area of PMF shadow in the coal-worker (Fig. 11). The contraction of areas of PMF causes a reduction in total lung capacity, except in old age when it may increase again with the extension of compensatory emphysema. The residual volume is typically increased both in absolute terms and as a percentage of total lung capacity. Lung compliance is usually reduced in young men in both complicated coal-workers' pneumoconiosis and silico-tuberculosis, but in the elderly compensatory emphysema may well increase it to above normal values. Exercise ventilation on breathing air may be slightly increased and the transfer factor for carbon monoxide is low both because the diffusing capacity of the alveolar capillary membrane is reduced and because there is usually a reduction in the volume of blood in the lung capillaries.

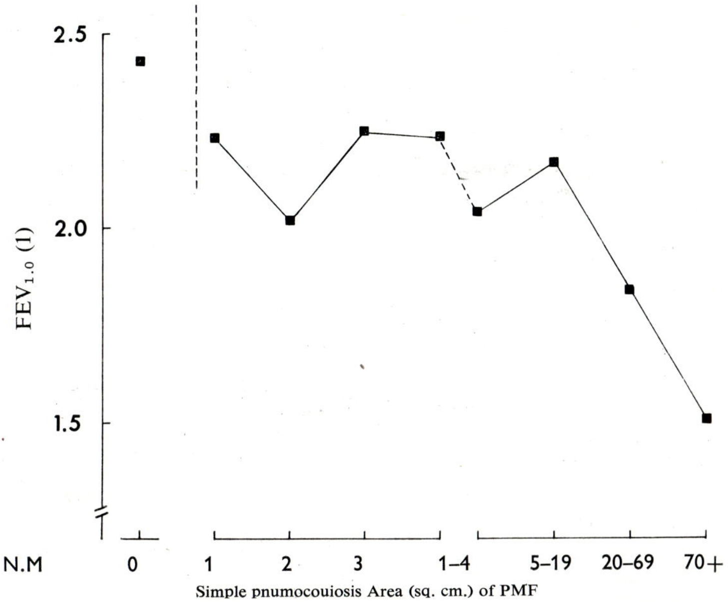

FIG. 11. The relation of ventilatory capacity ($FEV_{1 \cdot 0}$) to radiological category of simple pneumoconiosis and to the area of complicated pneumoconiosis (PMF) in miners and ex-miners age 55-64. A group of non-miners (N.M.) is also shown. (Cochrane et al, 1961.)

But exertional dyspnoea in progressive massive fibrosis is chiefly related to ventilatory impairment. The changes in ventilatory capacity vary widely; thus Gilson and Hugh-Jones (1955) found that the maximum voluntary ventilation of men with advanced progressive massive fibrosis was reduced to about one-third of normal. A useful review of lung function measurement is provided by the International Labour Office (1966).

Management

Coalworkers' Pneumoconiosis and Silicosis

Specific therapy. No means is known of influencing the retention or elimination of silica or coal-dust. Also there is no evidence that antituberculous chemotherapy or surgical excision affects the progression of complicated pneumoconiosis without tubercle bacilli in the sputum (Ball, Berry, Clarke, Gilson and Thomas, 1969). In cases with positive sputum, reversion is likely and the disease becomes quiescent on a standard regime of PAS and isoniazid, preferably with streptomycin initially.

The relationship between Caplan's syndrome and rheumatoid arthritis has suggested the possible value of penicillamine or other thiol compounds in its treatment, as these may dissociate polymeric rheumatoid factor molecules into inactive monomers by raising the protein sulphydryl levels, or act as chelating agents. Preliminary clinical evidence does not support the value of penicillamine in Caplan's syndrome, and serious side effects can occur.

In silicosis the possibility of influencing the action of silica dust once it is in the lung has been improved by the German discovery that the polymer polyvinyl-N-oxide (PNO) powerfully inhibits the fibrogenic action of silica both in tissue culture and in vivo. It acts by preventing silica particles from destroying the phagosome membrane of the phagocytic cells and may have considerable clinical value (see W.H.O., 1968).

Treatment of complications. Bronchitis often accompanies progressive massive fibrosis and exacerbations of infection need adequate chemotherapy. As a start, Ampicillin mg 500 four times daily for at least six days is usually more effective than a similar dose of a tetracycline. If the sputum purulence is not reduced in three days a culture should be taken and the antibiotic changed.

Pressurized inhalers containing isoprenaline or, preferably, salbutamol are useful in treating reversible bronchospasm, but oral antispasmodics such as the theophiline derivatives seem usually ineffective. Occasionally considerable improvement results from steroid therapy especially when there is sputum eosinophilia; serial measurements of ventilatory capacity are necessary to assess the response.

Congestive heart failure is treated by digitalization, diuretics and oxygen therapy as necessary. Unless facilities are available for the administration of controlled concentrations the oxygen flow should not exceed 2 l/min to avoid carbon dioxide narcosis.

At home the patient with severe disability should be encouraged to keep as mobile as possible, but to avoid sudden changes in temperature. Many men have found their mobility greatly increased by having their bed in the heated sitting room. Also an oxygen cylinder, preferably with a long tube to the face mask, can help a man to reach the lavatory, climb stairs, or perform other exertions of short duration. Small portable oxygen cylinders can be bought but cannot be prescribed on the National Health Service.

Advice on employment and compensation. The man with pneumoconiosis or silicosis needs advice on his work and on whether an application should be made to a Pneumoconiosis Panel for compensation under the National Insurance (Industrial Injuries) Act.

Suitable employment depends on his age, skills, the availability of alternative work and the stage of his disease. Every effort must be made to protect a man with pneumoconiosis from being exposed to concentrations of dust which are likely to cause further deterioration in his condition. However, it is not easy, except in the young man, or the older one with recent radiological deterioration, to judge whether his condition is due to dustier conditions in the past, particularly in the mining industry. The National Coal Board has made good progress in reducing the dust levels at its coal faces but special attention must be given to men who have already developed more than Category 1 pneumoconiosis. They should work in areas of a mine where the dust levels are low or should wear a dust filter mask when at the face. The possibility of an individual susceptibility must be considered in the case of young men with rapidly developing chest X-ray abnormalities and they should probably seek alternative work. Advice must include full discussion of the possibilities of other employment and men with any respiratory disability should be disuaded from entering an employment in which physical demands are close to their respiratory limit. Retraining in a Government Training Centre may be arranged. These number about thirty throughout the country and, subject to pretraining assessment, offer training in about forty trades, ranging from relatively heavy work such as bricklaying or engineering trades to light ones such as watch and clock repairing or tailoring. Any man, irrespective of age, who has no prospects of regular work in a skilled job may apply for assessment at a local office of the Ministry of Employment and Productivity.

Advice to the older man of 50 years or so will be tempered by the fact that many years' work has resulted in only a modest amount of disease, and the possibilities of alternative satisfactory employment are relatively limited.

In complicated pneumoconiosis there is no evidence that further dust exposure appreciably influences the rate of development of progressive massive fibrosis and advice on employment will be dictated chiefly by the prospect of further disability.

Compensation: Pneumoconiosis is defined at present under the National Insurance (Industrial Injuries) Act as "fibrosis of the lungs due to silica dust, asbestos dust or other dust and includes the condition known as dust reticulation." In practice the Pneumoconiosis Panels certify men as having pneumoconiosis if their chest X-ray shows an abnormality approximately equivalent to Category 2 or above. A man is eligible for consideration if at some time since 4th July, 1948 he has worked in one of a wide list of dusty occupations, the "scheduled occupations", or can satisfy the authorities that he has reasonable grounds for suspecting that he has pneumoconiosis. Special arrangements are made for those last employed in a dusty occupation before 5th July, 1948.

The applicant will have a chest X-ray at his nearest Pneumoconiosis Panel, and if it shows pneumoconiosis nearing Category 2 he will be recalled for medical examination to decide eligibility for compensation and its amount based on that proportion of disability thought to be due to pneumoconiosis. In addition an upward adjustment is made for the effects of certain other diseases such as bronchitis. The Panel will send the man a "letter of advice" saying whether he can safely continue work, and he is free to ignore this advice, unless he has tuberculosis, without his pension being affected. Subsequently his condition will be reviewed by the Pneumoconiosis Panel at intervals of one year or longer, and after his death a widow may be eligible for a pension.

References

Ashley, D. J. B. (1967), "The Distribution of Lung Cancer and Bronchitis in England and Wales." *Brit. J. Cancer*, **21,** 243.

Ball, J. D., Berry, G., Clarke, W. G., Gilson, J. C. and Thomas, J. (1969), "A Controlled Trial of Anti-tuberculosis Chemotherapy in the Early Complicated Pneumoconiosis of Coal-workers." *Thorax*, **24,** 399.

Bignall, J. C. (1969), Personal communication.

Brasseur, L. (1963), *L'exploration fonctionelle pulmonaire dans la pneumoconiose des houilleurs*. Brussels. Editions Arscia S.A.

Caplan, A. (1953), "Certain Unusual Radiological Appearances in the Chest of Coal-miners Suffering from Rheumatoid Arthritis." *Thorax*, **8,** 29.

Cochrane, A. L. (1962), "The Attack Rate of Progressive Massive Fibrosis." *Brit. J. Industr. Med.*, **19,** 52.

Cochrane, A. L., Higgins, I. T. T. and Thomas, J. (1961), "Pulmonary Ventilatory Functions of Coal-miners in Various Areas in Relation to the X-ray Category of Pneumoconiosis." *Brit. J Prev. Soc. Med.*, **15,** 1.

Englert, M. and De Coster, A. (1965), "La capacité de diffusion pulmonaire dans l'anthracosilicose micronodulaire." *J. Franç. Méd. Chir. Thor.*, **19,** 159.

Gilson, J. C. and Hugh-Jones, P. (1955), "Lung Function in Coal-workers' Pneumoconiosis." *Med. Res. Counc. Spec. Rep. Ser.*, No. 290.

Goldman, K. P. (1965), "Prognosis of Coal-miners with Cancer of the Lung." *Thorax*, **20,** 170.

Gough, J. (1947), "Pneumoconiosis in Coal-workers in Wales." *Occup. Med.*, **4,** 86.

Gye, W. E. and Kettle, E. H. (1922), "Silicosis and Miners' Phthisis." *Brit. J. Exp. Path.*, **3,** 241.

Harington, J. S. and Allison, A. C. (1965), "Lysosomal Enzymes in Relation to the Toxicity of Silica." *Med. del Lavoro*, **56,** 471.

Holt, P. F. (1957), *Pneumoconiosis*. London: Arnold.

International Labour Office (1959), "Meeting of Experts on the International Classification of Radiographs of the Pneumoconioses." *Occup. Safety Hlth.*, **9,** 2.

International Labour Office (1966), *Occupational Safety and Health series No. 6:* "Respiratory Function Tests in Pneumoconioses."

International Union Against Cancer Committee (1970), "UICC/Cincinnati Classification of Radiographic Appearances of Pneumoconioses." *Chest*, **58,** 57.

Jacobsen, M., Rae, S., Walton, W. H. and Rogan, J. M. (1971), "The Relation Between Pneumoconiosis and Dust Exposure in British Coal-miners." In *Inhaled Particles* III, p. 903. Ed. W. H. Walton. London: Unwin.

King, E. J., Zaidi, S. H. and Nagelschmidt, G. (1956), "The Silica-solubility Theory of Silicosis." *A.M.A. Arch. Industr. Hlth.*, **13,** 133.

Liddell, F. D. K. (1963), "An Experiment in Film Reading." *Brit. J. Industr. Med.*, **20,** 300.

Liddell, F. D. K. and May, Joan D. (1966), *Assessing the Radiological Progression of Simple Pneumoconiosis.* National Coal Board Medical Service (*Med. res. Memorandum No.* 4).

Lyons, J. P., Clark, W. G., Hall, A. M. and Cotes, J. E. (1967), "Transfer Factor (Diffusing Capacity) for the Lung in Simple Pneumoconiosis of Coal-workers." *Brit. Med. J.*, **4,** 772.

Marks, J., Mason, M. Ann and Nagelschmidt, G. (1956), "A Study of Dust Toxicity Using a Quantitative Tissue Culture Technique." *Brit. J. Industr. Med.*, **13,** 187.

McLintock, J. S., Rae, S. and Jacobsen, M. (1971), "The Attack Rate of Progressive Massive Fibrosis in British Coal-mines." In *Inhaled Particles* III, p. 933. Ed. W. H. Walton. London: Unwin.

Medical Research Council (1960), "Standardized Questionnaires on Respiratory Symptoms." *Brit. med. J.*, **2,** 1665.

Medical Research Council (1966), "Chronic Bronchitis and Occupation: Medical Research Council Report." *Brit. Med. J.*, **1,** 101.

Nagelschmidt, G. (1960), "A Review of Theories of Silicosis." In *A Symposium on Industrial Pulmonary Diseases.* Ed. by E. J. King and C. M. Fletcher, Ch. 5, p. 59. London: Churchill.

Rae, S., Walker, D. D. and Attfield, M. D. (1971), "Chronic Bronchitis and Dust Exposure in British Coal-miners." In *Inhaled Particles* III, p. 883. Ed. W. H. Walton. London: Unwin.

Registrar General (1951), *Registrar General's Decennial Supplement, England and Wales: Occupational Mortality, Part* 2, *Vol.* 1: *Commentary.* London: H.M.S.O., 1958.

Rivers, D., Wise, M. E., King, E. J. and Nagelschmidt, G. (1960), "Dust Content, Radiology and Pathology in Simple Pneumoconiosis of Coal-workers: Part 1. General Observations." *Brit. J. Industr. Med.*, **17,** 87.

Robock, K. (1967), "Die Messung der Lumineszenz verschiedener Siliciumdioxid-Modifikationen als Beitrag zur Frage der Silikoseentstehung." *Beitr. Silikose-Forsch.*, **92,** 1.

Rossiter, C. E., Rivers, D., Bergman, I., Casswell, C. and Nagelschmidt, G. (1966), "Dust Content, Radiology and Pathology in Simple Pneumoconiosis of Coal-workers (Further Report)." In *Inhaled Particles and Vapours* II. Ed. C. N. Davies, p. 419. Pergamon Press.

Vigliani, E. C. and Pernis, B. (1958), "Immunological Factors in the Pathogenesis of the Hyaline Tissue of Silicosis." *Brit. J. Industr. Med.*, **15,** 8.

Wagner, J. C. and McCormick, J. N. (1967), "Immunological Investigations of Coal-workers' Disease." *J. Roy. Coll. Phycns.*, **2,** 49.

Wise, M. E. and Oldham, P. D. (1963), "Estimating Progression of Coal-workers' Simple Pneumoconiosis from Readings of Radiological Categories." *Brit. J. Industr. Med.*, **20,** 124.

World Health Organization (1968), *Pneumoconiosis.* Report on a Symposium convened by the Regional Office for Europe of the World Health Organization, Copenhagen.

Chapter 8

Other Industrial Dusts

P. Lesley Bidstrup

Only those substances which, following inhalation in particulate form, cause lung disease will be discussed (see Table 1). It should be remembered that many other systems may be affected by toxic substances

Table 1

Summary of conditions described

Condition	*Substance*	*Name of disease*
Radio-opaque shadows: no disability	Barium sulphate	Baritosis
	Cerium fluoride	—
	Iron oxide	Siderosis
	Tin oxide (lode ore) or dioxide (smelting)	Stannosis
	Titanium dioxide	Titanosis
	Cement dust	—
Bronchospasm and pneumonitis	Beryllium	Acute beryllium disease
	Cadmium oxide	Acute cadmium pneumonitis
	Vanadium pentoxide	—
	Hexavalent chromium compounds	—
	Hydrofluoric acid and complex fluorides	—
	Zinc chloride	—
	Volatile boron hydrides	—
Fibrosis	Aluminium dust	—
	Bauxite	Shaver's disease
	? Cobalt	Hard metal disease
	Haematite	Silico-siderosis
	Talc	Talcosis
Granulomatosis	Beryllium	Chronic beryllium disease
	Hair spray lacquers	Thesaurosis Hair spray lacquer disease
	Animal oils	Oleo-granuloma
	Mineral oils	Paraffinoma
Emphysema	Cadmium oxide	Chronic cadmium poisoning
Metal fume fever	Oxides of many metals, particularly zinc, copper, manganese	Metal fume fever

Table 1 (*Continued*)

Condition	*Substance*	*Name of disease*
Polymer fume fever	Thermal decomposition of polytetrafluoroethylene 'Teflon' 'Fluon'	Polymer fume fever
Carcinoma	Established causes:	
	Radioactive dusts	Carcinoma of lung
	Manufacture of bichromates	Carcinoma of lung
	Refining of nickel by decomposition of a gaseous nickel compound	Carcinoma of lung and nasal sinuses
	Dust of arsenic and compounds	Carcinoma of lung and nasal sinuses
	Asbestos dust	Carcinoma of lung Mesothelioma
	Manufacture of coal gas (obsolete process)	Carcinoma of lung
	Mining of haematite	Carcinoma of lung
	Hardwood Dust	Adenocarcinoma of nasal cavities
	Suspected causes:	
	Manufacture of isopropyl alcohol (obsolete process)	Carcinoma of lung and nasal sinuses
	Dust arising in iron and steel foundries, boiler-scaling and sand blasting	Carcinoma of lung
	Manufacture of chrome pigments	Carcinoma of lung

which enter the body through the respiratory tract. Examples are the effects of lead, manganese and mercury—inhaled as dust particles or vapour—pesticides, particularly when formulated as wettable powders or dust formulations, and the bladder carcinogens benzidine, α-β-naphthylamine, 4-amino-diphenyl and 4-nitro-diphenyl. Textbooks on occupational diseases should be consulted for descriptions of systemic disease of occupational origin.

1. **Inert dusts**

The inhalation of dust of fine particle size may result in deposition in the lung tissue of radio-opaque material which does not cause fibrosis or other tissue reaction. On X-ray examination opacities, the size and clarity of which depend upon the amount of dust present and on the atomic weight, are seen scattered evenly throughout the lung fields. The patient has no symptoms referable to the respiratory system, nor are there any abnormal signs present. Examples are—

(1) **Baritosis**—due to inhalation of barium sulphate (baryta) when mining, crushing, grinding or packing baryta (Fig. 1).

(2) **Cerium fluoride**—is obtained from monazite sand, the source of rare earth metals and oxides. It is used in the arc carbon and metallurgical industries. Grinding and sifting operations may be particularly dusty (Fig. 2).

(3) **Siderosis**—results from inhalation of iron or iron-oxide dust to which welders, haematite miners, mirror polishers and silver polishers may be exposed (Doig and McLaughlin, 1936; McLaughlin *et al.*, 1945).

(4) **Stannosis**—due to inhalation of tin oxide present in the lode ore of tin mines in Bolivia and Cornwall, and tin dioxide which occurs as dust or fume in the refining processes (Robertson, 1964).

(5) **Titanosis**—from dust of titanium dioxide used as a white pigment in paints, varnishes and lacquers.

(6) **Cement dust**—diagnosis is made from the occupational history, and the absence of symptoms and signs, despite the impressive radiological appearances.

2. **Bronchospasm and Pneumonitis**

Lung irritation characterized by bronchospasm, and often moist sounds, may follow exposure to a number of metals, or compounds of metals, in finely-divided form. Cough and dyspnoea, often accompanied by retrosternal pain or discomfort, are the presenting symptoms. There is usually a latent interval, which may be as long as 48 hours, between exposure and the onset of symptoms. There may be no X-ray changes and unless a careful occupational history is taken, the cause of the symptoms and signs may be overlooked. In such cases, the patient may be put at further risk by being allowed to resume work in an unsafe environment and others engaged in similar work will continue to be at risk.

Examples are—

(1) Acute beryllium disease—exposure to beryllium, or beryllium oxide, may occur in—
- (a) the extraction of the metal from the ore
- (b) the manufacture of alloys containing beryllium
- (c) the metallurgical processing of pure beryllium
- (d) the use of beryllium in research and development of atomic energy and space exploration projects.
- (e) the manufacture of radio-tubes, neon signs or ceramics containing beryllium
- (f) the manufacture and use of beryllium-containing coatings for fluorescent lamps (an obsolete process).

It is possible, also, that processes in which alloys containing beryllium are used, may present a hazard. These are processes where the temperature of the alloy may be raised to above the melting point (1,100°F) as in welding in open atmosphere or where grinding and similar operations are carried out without efficient exhaust ventilation or dust suppression with water.

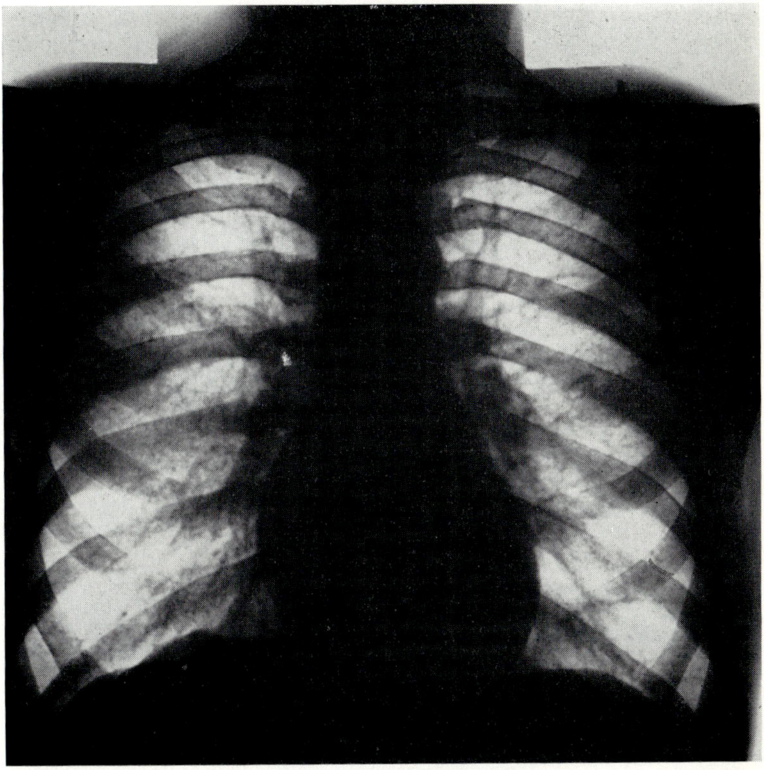

FIG. 1. WJTG: Exposure to dust of barium sulphate in pigment manufacture.

Disabling dyspnoea, cough, cyanosis and rapid weight loss are features of the disease which may prove fatal or be followed by the chronic form of the disease (see page 164) immediately or after a latent interval of many years during which the patient is free from symptoms. In the majority of patients, recovery is complete within one to six months.

Diagnosis depends on the history of exposure to beryllium and the use of the stethoscope. The X-ray may show diffuse bilateral haziness, increased peri-bronchial markings, soft irregular areas of infiltration, and at a later stage discrete large or small nodules (Tepper, Hardy and Chamberlain, 1961). There may, however, be no X-ray changes in a patient who is seriously disabled by the disease (Fig. 3). Treatment is symptomatic but it is thought that steroids may lessen the impact of the disease and shorten its course. Bed rest, and when necessary, the administration of oxygen, are essential features of treatment.

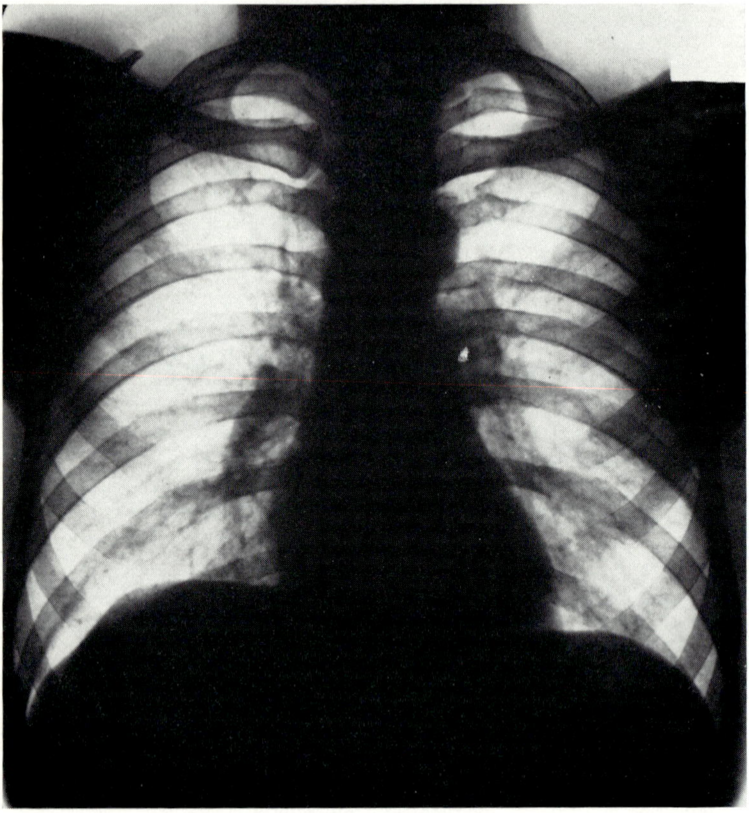

FIG. 2. AST: Exposure to dust of cerium fluoride. No symptoms or signs. Appearance unchanged over 25 years.

(2) **Cadmium fume**—is generated from molten cadmium during smelting, in the manufacture of alloys, in "metalizing" with cadmium, and in the cutting or welding of cadmium-coated metals. Pulmonary oedema has resulted from such work carried out in confined spaces or inadequately ventilated workshops.

Symptoms include intense, burning pain behind the sternum, violent cough, vomiting and dyspnoea. There may be no X-ray changes, but in some cases hilar congestion and diffuse soft shadows in both lungs are observed (Evans, 1960; Karlish, 1960; Kleinfield, Messite and Giel, 1958).

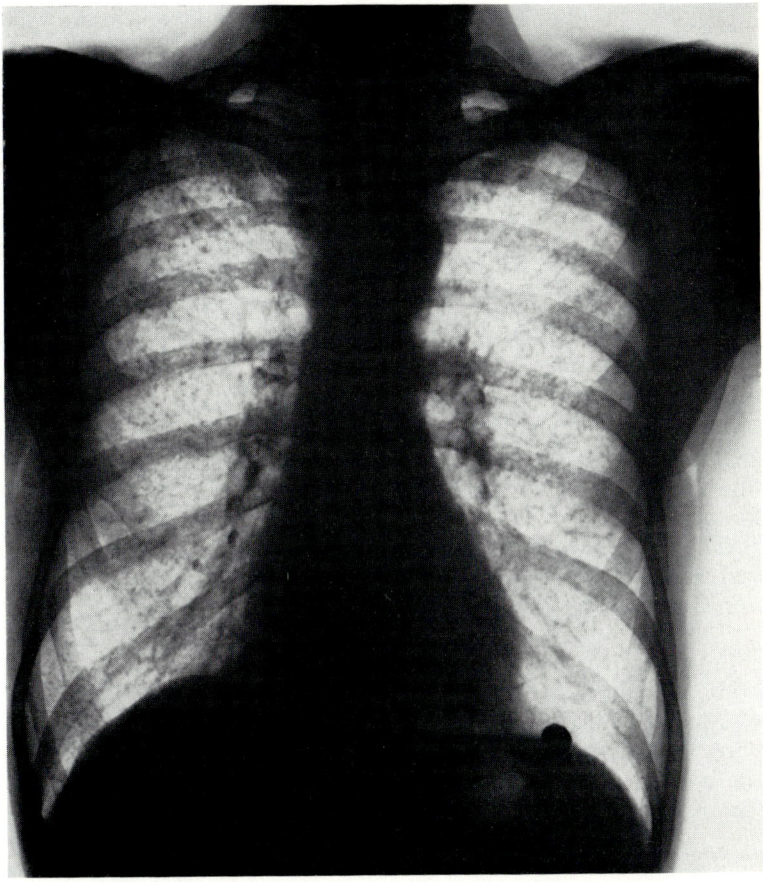

FIG. 3. JB: Acute beryllium disease. Patient seriously disabled. Moist sounds all areas—no X-ray changes.

Treatment is symptomatic and recovery complete within a few weeks. There are no sequelae but repeated inhalation of less irritant concentrations results in chronic cadmium poisoning (see page 169).

(3) **Vanadium pentoxide**—is used for metallurgical purposes and as a catalyst in many chemical processes. It is also deposited in flues, stacks, heat-exchange pipes and firebrick walls of boilers when fuel oils having a high vanadium content are burnt in furnaces firing boilers to raise

steam for ships or to provide heat for industrial processes. Men engaged in cleaning flues and boilers are at risk of inhaling dust containing vanadium pentoxide.

It is very irritating to the mucous membranes of the eyes, nose, throat and smaller air passages causing bronchospasm and sometimes moist sounds in the lungs. There are usually no X-ray changes. A green or black discoloration of the tongue may assist in diagnosis (Lewis, 1959).

Treatment is symptomatic and there are no sequelae.

(4) **Hexavalent chromium**—dust or mist containing hexavalent chromium will cause ulceration of the nasal septum followed by perforation. When the edges of the perforation are healed the condition is usually symptom free and many persons who have perforation of the nasal septum are unaware of it.

Bronchospasm may follow inhalation of high concentrations producing a condition indistinguishable clinically from bronchitis but of short duration. A few people become sensitized and must be removed from further risk of exposure.

(5) Other substances which may produce bronchospasm or pneumonitis are *hydrofluoric acid* and *complex compounds of fluorine* arising when a water-based fluoride flux is used in the jointing of high-tension cables (Bonnell, personal communication); these fluxes may contain aminoethylethanolamine which is a potent sensitizing agent: *zinc chloride* used as a smoke-screen and the *volatile boron hydrides* used as rocket propellants.

3. Pulmonary Fibrosis

(1) **Aluminium dust**—there is no doubt that dust of aluminium powder of respirable particle size will cause interstitial fibrosis of the lungs. The effects were described first in Germany in 1938 and cases have been reported subsequently in Sweden, Japan and Great Britain. All have occurred among persons at risk of inhaling finely-divided aluminium powder, known as "pyro", which is used in fireworks or mixed with explosives; a coarser powder used in aluminium paint may cause X-ray changes of less severity and without associated symptoms. Some authorities, however, regard aluminium dust as harmless and it has been used in the prevention and treatment of silicosis.

The literature is reviewed and cases described by Mitchell and his colleagues (1961). These arose in the preparation of aluminium powders. Jordan (1961) reports on the disease in a young woman who had filled fireworks with a mixture of aluminium powder and potassium perchlorate, and McLaughlin *et al.* (1962) record a case in which central nervous system effects dominated the clinical picture.

Although clinical and radiological evidence of lung involvement in this patient was slight, post-mortem examination revealed fibrosis, particularly in the upper lobes, and confirmed the presence of aluminium dust in the lungs. Under refracted light aluminium flakes about 20 μg across could be seen which were similar in size and shape to the dust collected in the factory. The aerodynamic size of these flakes was such that they could penetrate to the alveoli.

The presenting symptom is dyspnoea, which progresses rapidly. X-ray changes include fine granular or coarser opacities, particularly in the upper and middle zones, displacement upwards of the hilar shadows with widening of the mediastinum and deviation of the trachea to the right. Elevation and tenting of the diaphragm is common, and in some cases, spontaneous pneumothorax occurs as a late complication.

The disease resembles in many respects the condition described by Shaver and Riddell (1947) due to inhalation of the fumes arising during the calcining of *bauxite*. In this process, however, silica is also present whereas the patients referred to above were exposed only to aluminium.

(2) **Hard Metal disease**—Bech, Kipling and Heather (1962) describe pulmonary fibrosis in six among 255 men employed in the hard-metal (*tungsten carbide*) industry. The metal is produced by powder metallurgy from tungsten and carbon using cobalt as a binder. The cutting edges of tools, rock drills, broaches and dies are made from hard metal which is used also for radiotherapy screens and armaments. In the manufacturing process dust may be produced during mixing, filtering and shaping of the powders and in grinding operations.

The cause of the disease is not known but Bech and his colleagues suggest that the component of the dust which may be responsible is *cobalt*. Their investigation indicates that the disease is not common among those at risk, cases tending to occur sporadically. There may be few symptoms in relation to the X-ray changes, but when present include productive cough, dyspnoea and tightness in the chest.

The X-ray changes are prominent hilar shadows, exaggerated linear markings and micro-nodular opacities widely distributed throughout the lungs but particularly in the mid and lower zones. In a fatal case diffuse interstitial fibrosis and marked peribronchial and perivascular fibrosis were found.

(3) **Haematite**—although the dust of haematite is composed largely of iron oxide, the ore mined in Cumberland contains 10% of silica and is dry, crystalline and very hard. In these respects it differs from the ferric oxide or haematite, which is used in silver polishing, or which arises from electric welding, boiler scaling, metal grinding and fettling. Faulds (1957) describes haematite pneumonoconiosis, which is a sidero-silicosis, found in Cumberland miners. Effects on the lungs of haematite miners were rare until 1930, the increased incidence observed at that time being

due to the introduction, in 1913 of pneumatic drilling to replace hand drilling. The pneumatic drill produced a voluminous cloud of dust of fine particle size which was blown back into the miner's face by compressed air.

In contrast to the small widely scattered opacities found in siderosis, the lesion in sidero-silicosis, is one of progressive massive fibrosis involving extensive areas of the lungs. The hard fibrotic tissue coalesces and is coloured brick-red by the haematite. Dust suppression measures were introduced in the late 1930s and the incidence of the disease has diminished. The X-ray reveals scattered small opacities with areas of massive shadowing mainly in the upper zones.

(4) **Talc**—Talc is a double silicate of magnesium but in contrast with asbestos is composed of plates with only a few fibres. Long exposure to talc results in fibrosis of the lungs affecting mainly the lower lobes.

McLaughlin *et al.* (1949) described the histological appearances in a case of talc pneumonoconiosis in a man who had worked for 37 years in a rubber tyre factory where he had been exposed to talc dust for long periods. Small grey nodules were scattered throughout the lung substance but were more numerous in the lower lobes. There were, in addition, "talc" bodies resembling, but easily distinguishable from asbestos bodies.

4. **Granulomatous lesions**

(1) **Beryllium (Chronic beryllium disease)**—The sources of exposure to beryllium or beryllium oxide, from which chronic beryllium disease may result, are the same as those listed under "Acute beryllium disease" (see page 158).

Acute beryllium disease may progress to the chronic form without remission. In many cases, however, the chronic disease develops years after an acute episode, the patient having been symptom free and having had no further exposure to beryllium during the latent period. It may occur also in persons who have been working with beryllium or its compounds but in whom there is no history of an acute episode. It may arise while the patient is still exposed to beryllium, or many years after the last known exposure.

The disease is characterized by marked shortness of breath, loss of weight and non-productive cough. Other systems, including the liver and kidneys, may be involved and in some cases skin lesions indistinguishable from those of sarcoidosis are seen. The condition may be totally disabling, but in many cases remissions occur. Diffuse granular or nodular opacities occur throughout the lungs with enlargement of the hilar shadows due, probably, to enlargement of the pulmonary vessels. The radiological appearances are similar to those of sarcoid

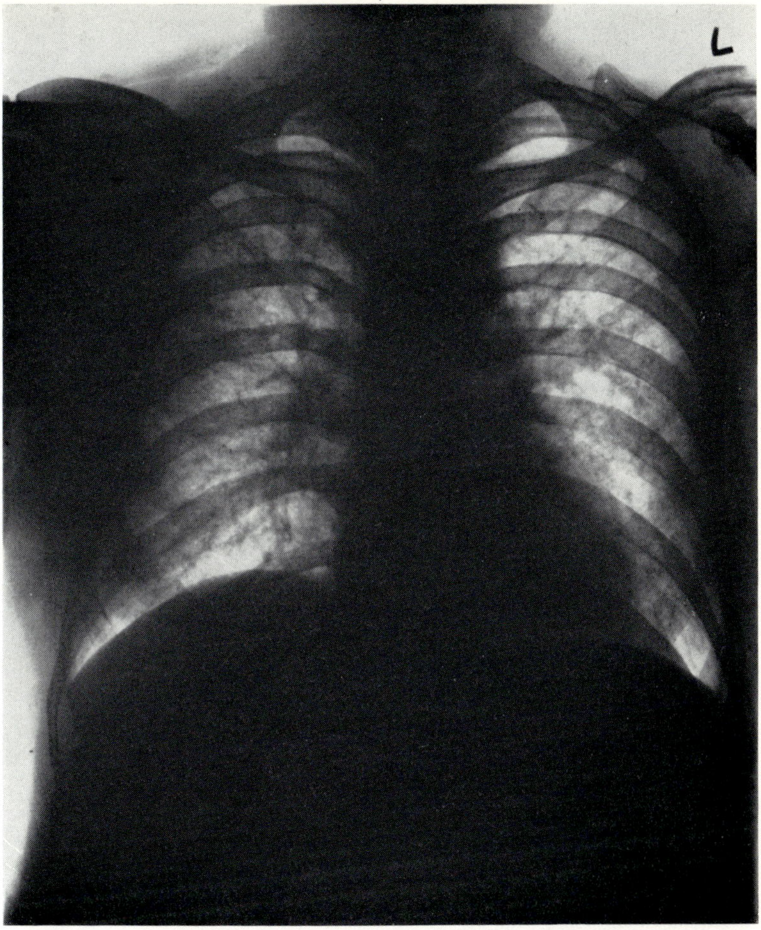

FIG. 4. CRB: Chronic beryllium disease, 15 March, 1951. Exposure to fluorescent lamp powders containing beryllium—1942–7. No further exposure but in 1951 developed symptoms, signs and X-ray evidence of chronic beryllium disease.

(Fig. 4). They are due to granulomatous infiltration in septal, subpleural, perivascular and peribronchial tissues and involve both lungs diffusely. There is also chronic inflammatory infiltration and inclusion body formation within giant cells. Contraction due to fibrosis and compensatory emphysema complicate the clinical and X-ray pictures in the later stages of the disease (Fig. 5). The reader is referred to the monograph on the toxicity of beryllium compounds by Tepper, Hardy and Chamberlain (1961).

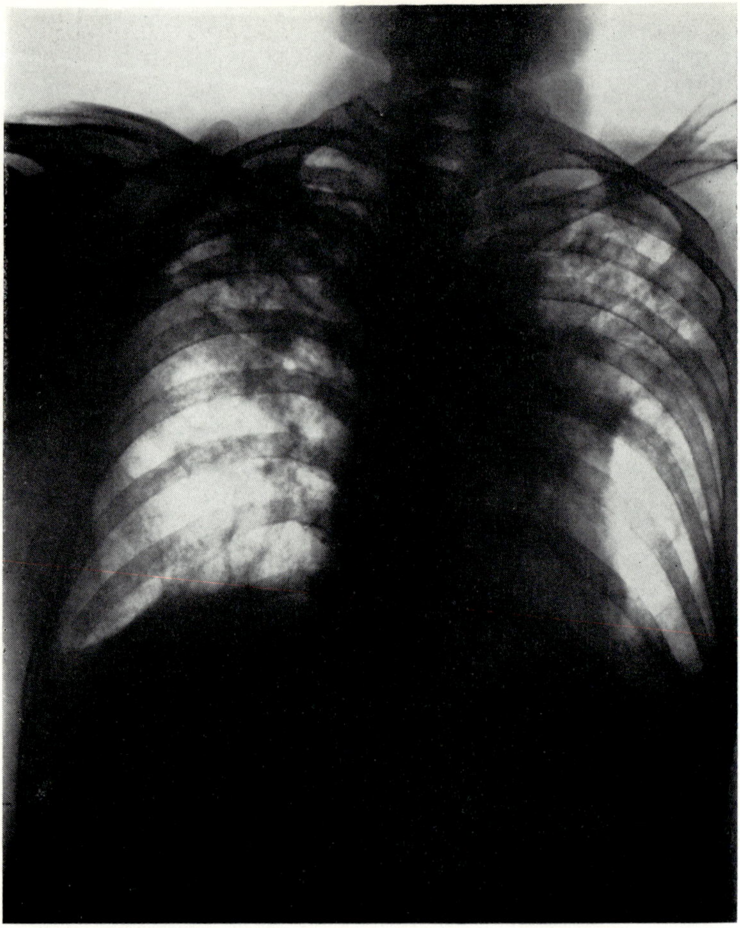

FIG. 5. CRB: Chronic beryllium disease, 2 January, 1956. Film taken in 1956 shortly before death shows scarring and contraction with compensatory emphysema and displacement of mediastinum.

Differential diagnosis—particularly from sarcoidosis, miliary tuberculosis and lymphangitic carcinomatosis—may be difficult. It depends upon the history of exposure to berryllium or its compounds and the X-ray changes. Moist sounds at the bases of the lung may be heard but often there are no signs. The presence of beryllium in the urine is evidence of exposure to beryllium but is not necessarily diagnostic. Lung biopsy may reveal the classical histological picture and the presence of beryllium in lung tissue. Lung function tests demonstrate the typical findings associated with disease of the lung parenchyma.

The transfer factor for carbon monoxide is reduced and the ventilation on exercise is increased. Airway obstruction is not a feature. The total lung volume and the compliance of the lungs are reduced. Arterial desaturation occurs as the disease progresses and may fall further on exercise. The carbon dioxide tension of the arterial blood is either normal or reduced. Treatment is symptomatic but should include the administration of steroids which frequently alleviate the symptoms but do not alter the X-ray appearances.

(2) **Lacquer hair sprays**—Two types of lacquer, one shellac-based and the other containing polyvinyl-pyrrolidone (PVP), are used by women's hairdressers and by individual women and sometimes men, in their homes. In 1958, Bergmann and his colleagues drew attention to the fact that the use of either type of lacquer may cause diffuse pulmonary fibrosis accompanied by hilar lymphadenopathy. Since that time there have appeared other case reports indicating the potential risk of using lacquer hair sprays. It is likely that the reaction occurs only in susceptible or hypersensitive people, since very few cases have been reported despite the extensive use of lacquer hair sprays in hairdressing salons and by millions of individuals, often daily.

McLaughlin *et al.* (1963) found no cases among 458 hairdressers investigated by clinical and X-ray examination, but in the course of the survey one case of interstitial pulmonary fibrosis in a woman exposed to shellac-based hair sprays for eleven years was brought to the attention of the investigators. It was shown in this survey that the majority of particles from both hand sprays and pressure aerosol sprays were less than 1 μ in diameter.

The condition is known as *thesaurosis* but *hair spray lacquer disease* is a more acceptable name. On X-ray opacities are seen throughout both lungs and the hilar glands are enlarged. In many cases the X-ray changes disappear when the practice of using lacquer hair sprays is discontinued (Figs. 6 and 7).

(3) **Oils**—Kazantzis (1961) in a report on air contamination arising from the use of high speed dental drills, found no evidence of risk of lung damage from oil spray to dentist or patient, but reviews the literature relating to the harmful effects of oil on the lungs.

A granulomatous tissue reaction with surrounding fibrosis may occur and has been named *oleo-granuloma.* Inhalation of *animal oils* produces an inflammatory reaction characterized by the presence of many multi-nucleated foreign body giant cells and large mono-nuclear cells with oil-laden cytoplasm. In children who have inhaled, for example, cod-liver oil, acute pneumonic consolidation, which resolves, has been observed.

Mineral oil induces a slower but intense fibrous tissue reaction surrounding collections of oil-laden macrophages. Firm masses develop which may resemble carcinoma and are known as *paraffinoma*. Such lesions have occurred following inhalation of liquid paraffin administered for medicinal reasons. By contrast, vegetable oils are apparently

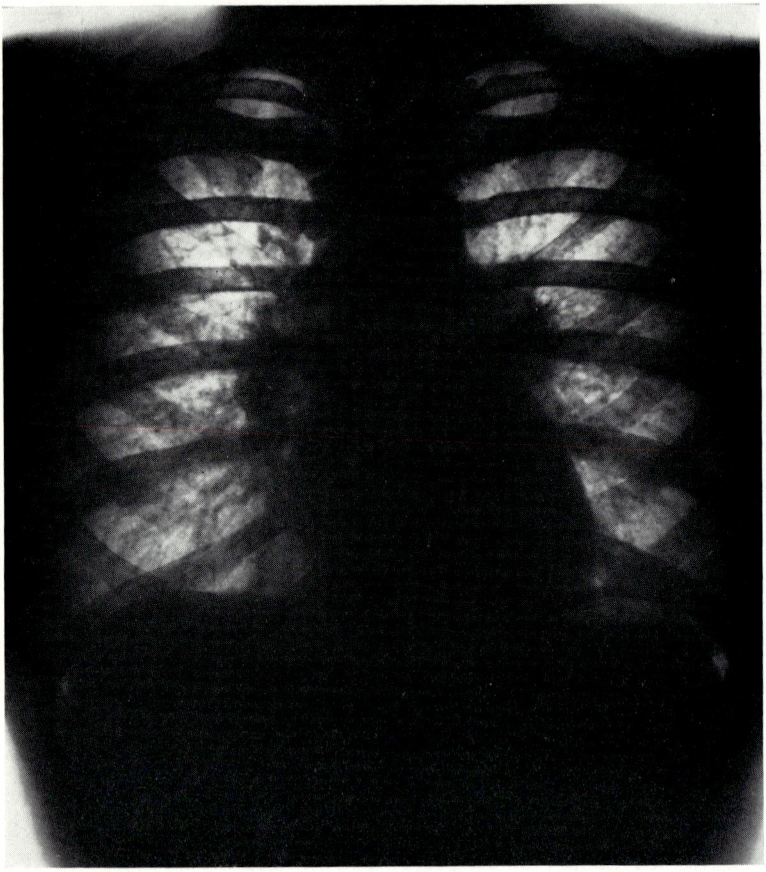

FIG. 6. MB: ? Hair spray lacquer disease, 17 July, 1964. Referred from MMR. Symptom free. "Beehive" hair style.

harmless, iodized vegetable oil being used frequently in contrast radiology of the lungs.

These pathological lesions have only been described following gross inhalation of liquid oils. No clinical cases of lung damage following the inhalation of oil droplets or aerosol have been described. Many industrial workers are exposed to compressed air which may be contaminated with oil and a careful watch must be maintained.

(5) **Emphysema (Chronic cadmium poisoning).** The inhalation of dust or fume containing *cadmium oxide* or *salts of cadmium* in concentrations insufficient to cause acute respiratory illness, gives rise to emphysema of

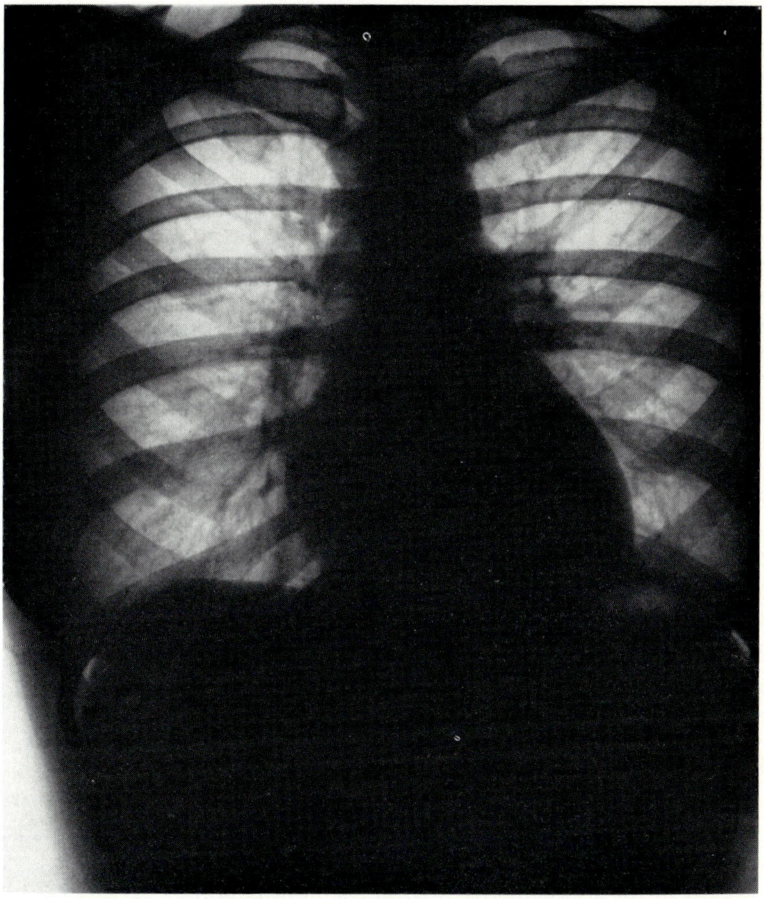

FIG. 7. MB: Five months later, 18 December, 1964. X-ray normal. No further use of lacquer hair sprays.

insidious onset, associated, usually with renal tubular damage manifested by the presence in the urine of a protein of low molecular weight. The disease is known as CHRONIC CADMIUM poisoning (Bonnell, 1955).

The onset of symptoms is gradual and may or may not be preceded by irritation of the nose and throat and loss of sense of smell. Unusual fatigue and shortness of breath are the usual presenting symptoms. The clinical and X-ray findings are characteristic of emphysema of unknown aetiology. Unlike the emphysema which follows asthma or bronchitis of long duration, the dyspnoea of chronic cadmium poisoning precedes, often by several years, the onset of troublesome cough. This fact is helpful in differential diagnosis. The presence of protein in the urine which may not be precipitated by boiling but is demonstrated by using 25 % trichloracetic acid or 3 % sulpho-salicylic acid in the cold, together with a history of exposure to cadmium compounds in respirable form, confirms the diagnosis of chronic cadmium poisoning. Emphysema may, however, precede the proteinuria.

(6) **Metal fume fever.** Molten metals may give off a vapour which, on cooling in air, condenses to form a fine aerosol or fume of oxide particles. The individual particles may be smaller than 0·1 micron in diameter but they are always aggregated into complex chains. The fumes of many metals, and particularly those of zinc, copper and manganese cause illnesses resembling influenza but of shorter duration.

The symptoms begin some hours after exposure. Intense headache, aching of muscles and rigors characterize the clinical picture. There may be a slight rise in temperature and there is an associated leucocytosis. There are no X-ray changes. The symptoms subside within 12–24 hours leaving a feeling of weakness but no sequlae.

It is thought that the illness is due to deposition of fine particles of metal oxide in the lung combining with tissue protein to cause an antigen–antibody reaction. Some immunity is acquired on continued exposure but this is lost during short absences from work and the symptoms recur on re-exposure.

A similar condition results from the thermal decomposition of polytetrafluoro-ethylene ("Fluon"; "Teflon") or from finely-divided dust and is called polymer fume fever.

(7) **Carcinoma of lung and nasal sinuses.** Epidemiological and statistical investigations have shown that the incidence of lung cancer among men engaged in the following occupations is unusually high—

(1) Work involving exposure to radioactive dusts.
(2) The refining of nickel by decomposition of a gaseous nickel compound (Lung and nasal sinuses).
(3) Exposure to asbestos dust.
(4) The manufacture of chromates from the ore, chromite.
(5) The manufacture of coal gas by a process which is becoming obsolete.
(6) The mining of haematite.
(7) Exposure to arsenic and its compounds (Lung and nasal sinuses).

(8) Adenocarcinoma of the nasal cavities has been shown by Acheson *et al.* (1968) to occur in workers making furniture from hard woods such as oak or beech. The authors consider that the association is due to the inhalation of wood particles.

There may be a similar risk associated with an obsolete process for the manufacture of isopropyl alcohol (lung and nasal sinuses); among men working in iron and steel foundries; in boiler-scaling and in sandblasting; and in the manufacture of chrome pigments.

The processes concerned are described and the epidemiological and statistical evidence presented by Raven (1960) and Raven and Roe (1967).

The clinical features of lung and nasal cancer of occupational origin are no different from those of cancer of unknown aetiology occurring at these sites. The disease may not develop until many years—commonly about 20—after exposure to the hazard, and the symptoms may not appear until after a man has retired from work, or changed to an occupation which is considered to be free of any particular risk to health. It is therefore important to record a full occupational history in all cases. Cancer of occupational origin usually occurs at an earlier age than cancer of unknown aetiology arising at similar sites. Multiple primary tumours tend also to be a feature of cancer of occupational origin.

Diagnosis depends on frequent X-ray and clinical examination of men who are likely to be affected. The value of exfoliative cytology remains to be established but is worth undertaking in cases of persistent cough or recurrent bronchitis. No tests are known at present which make it possible to distinguish lung or nasal cancer of occupational origin from similar cases in which the aetiology is unknown.

References

Acheson, E. D., Cowdell, R. H., Hadfield, E. and MacBeth, R. G. (1968), *Brit. Med. J.*, **1**, 587–96.

Bech, A. D., Kipling, M. D. and Heather, J. C. (1962), "Hard Metal Disease." *Brit. J. Ind. Med.*, **19**, 239.

Bergman, M., Flance, I. J. and Blumenthal, H. T. (1958), "Thesaurosis Following Inhalation of Hair Spray." *New Eng. J. Med.*, **258**, 471.

Bonnell, J. A. (1955), "Emphysema and Proteinuria in Men Casting Copper-cadmium Alloys." *Brit. J. Ind. Med.*, **12**, 181.

Doig, A. T. and McLaughlin, A. I. G. (1936), "X-ray Appearances of the Lungs of Electric Arc Welders." *Lancet*, **1**, 771.

Evans, D. M. (1960), "Cadmium Poisoning." *Brit. Med. J.*, **1**, 173.

Faulds, J. S. (1957), "Haematite Pneumoconiosis in Cumberland Miners." *J. Clin. Path.*, **10**, 187.

Jordan, J. W. (1961), "Pulmonary Fibrosis in a Worker Using an Aluminium Powder." *Brit. J. Ind. Med.*, **12**, 21.

Karlish, A. J. (1960), "Cadmium Poisoning." *Brit. Med. J.*, **1**, (corresp.), 727.

Kazantzis, G. (1961), "Air Contamination from High Speed Dental Drills." *Proc. Roy. Soc. Med.*, **54**, 242.

Kleinfield, M., Messite, J. and Giel, C. P. (1958), "Pulmonary Oedema of Non-cardiac Origin." *Amer. J. Med. Sci.*, **235,** 660.

Lewis, C. E. (1959), "The Biological Effects of Vanadium." *A.M.A. Arch. Envir. Hlth.*, **19,** 497.

McLaughlin, A. I. G., Bidstriup, P. L. and Konstam, M. (1963), "The Effects of Hair Lacquer Sprays on the Lungs." *Fd. Cosmet. Toxical.*, **1,** 171.

McLaughlin, A. I. G., Group, J. L. A., Barrie, H. J. and Harding, H. E. (1945), "Iron Oxide Dust and the Lungs of Silver Finishers." *Lancet*, **1,** 337.

McLaughlin, A. I. G., Kazantzis, G., King, E., Teare, D., Porter, R. J. and Owen, R. (1962), "Pulmonary Fibrosis and Encephalopathy Associated with the Inhalation of Aluminium Dust." *Brit. J. Ind. Med.*, **19,** 253.

McLaughlin, A. I. G., Rogers, E. and Dunham, K. C. (1949), "Talc Pneumoconiosis." *Brit. J. Ind. Med.*, **6,** 184.

Mitchell, J., Manning, G. B., Molyneux, M. and Lane, R. E. (1961), "Pulmonary Fibrosis in Workers Exposed to Finely Powdered Aluminium." *Brit. J. Ind. Med.*, **18,** 10.

Raven, R. W. (Ed.) (1960), In *Cancer Progress*, p. 81. London: Butterworth.

Raven, R. W. and Roe, F. J. C. (Ed.) (1967), In *The Prevention of Cancer*, p. 193. London: Butterworth.

Robertson, A. J. (1964), "The Romance of Tin." *Lancet*, **1,** 1229 and 1289.

Shaver, C. G. and Riddell, A. R. (1947), "Lung Changes Associated with the Manufacture of Aluminium Abrasives." *J. Ind. Hyg. and Toxicol.*, **29,** 145.

Tepper, L. B., Hardy, H. L. and Chamberlain, R. I. (1961), *Toxicity of Beryllium Compounds*, pp. 30–39. Elsevier Pub. Co.

Chapter 9

Physical Properties of Therapeutic Aerosols

D. C. F. MUIR

The importance attached to aerosol therapy by physicians and anaesthetists in different countries varies widely. Some hospitals support elaborate departments where, for example, antibiotics are routinely administered by the inhalation route for the treatment of pulmonary diseases while physicians at other centres feel that the various techniques have only a very limited part to play. No doubt these different views reflect the difficulty of assessing the clinical results since the immediate benefit obtained from bronchodilator aerosols is much less obvious in such instances as sputum liquifiers or mist tent therapy. The same problem arises in considering the real importance of the optimum size and composition of the particles. Measurement of the particle size in a liquid spray presents formidable problems and reliable information on the characteristics of a particular nebulizer is seldom available. Even when this is known there is no method at present of predicting the site of particle deposition in the diseased lung with any certainty. With these reservations the general principles underlying the techniques of aerosol therapy are reviewed in this chapter but no attempt is made to discuss the pharmacology of individual compounds.

Bronchodilator Aerosols

The inhalation of atropine from the smoke of burning stramonium leaves has been used for centuries in the treatment of asthma, and atropine cigarettes are still occasionally used. Particles produced by combustion in this way are usually exceedingly small (0·1–0·4 μ diameter). They are probably about the same size as those of tobacco smoke, although no measurements have been published. Ephraim (1910) first suggested the topical application of adrenaline solutions and this was followed by many reports in the German literature on the treatment of respiratory disorders by means of atomizers. Various forms of nebulizers were produced by commercial firms and advertised directly in the lay press. Greaser and Rowe (1935) reviewed the available patterns and studied their use for the inhalation of adrenaline. Before starting their experiments they had supposed that atomizers were simply a method of avoiding the use of injections. They thought that the inhaled drug would be absorbed from the mucosa into the blood stream and exert its effect as when given by injection. They were immediately struck by the speed of action of inhaled adrenaline and by the fact that it was possible to obtain relief of bronchospasm without the same degree of side effects such as tachycardia that were so common when it was given by injection. They concluded that the observed effects were due to a local action and recommended that atomizers should be designed to give small droplets since these were more likely to penetrate into the lung. Much ingenuity has been expended since then on the production of nebulizers reputed to give clouds of optimal particle size. The difficulty of knowing where the particles are, in fact, deposited is further complicated by disagreement as to the desired site of deposition. Most authors have felt that the important site of action is in the small bronchi and bronchioles where there is a plentiful supply of smooth muscle and which is known to be hypertrophied in asthma. It is generally considered that the aim of bronchodilator therapy should be to achieve a high concentration of the pharmacological agent in these regions, with a minimum deposition of particles in the mouth and larger airways where they can have no beneficial local action, and more likely to increase the unwanted side effects on the heart. Segal (1962) also suggested that particles small enough to penetrate to the alveoli should be avoided if possible since they could have no beneficial effect at those sites.

A different view of the action of inhaled bronchodilators was taken by Dautrebande (1962). He agreed that the incidence of undesirable side effects was related to the total absorbed dose, but considered that the local effects depended on the number of sites of action of the drug and hence on the actual number of inhaled particles. This observation was based on the fact that only one or two inhalations of bronchodilator aerosols containing a high concentration of particles produced as much improvement in asthmatic subjects as 20 or 30 such inhalations. Dautrebande also thought it desirable to achieve the deposition of particles in the alveolar regions of the lung. The alveolar ducts are known to be well supplied with muscle fibres and, in his view, this fact has been neglected in assessing the pathogenesis of asthma. Evidence that contraction of these fibres can, indeed, cause marked constriction of the alveolar ducts with associated changes in lung compliance was obtained by Nadel *et al.* (1967) who examined histological preparations of cat lungs following the inhalation of fine particles of histamine.

It is difficult to obtain experimental evidence to support the supposition that bronchodilator aerosols of a particular size produce relatively more bronchodilation, but fewer side effects, than clouds containing larger or smaller particles. Much confusion has arisen because of failure to allow for the fact that the size of the particles in a cloud usually governs the total absorbed dose of a pharmacological agent as well as the site of its deposition in the lung. A further factor is that the response of patients with asthma to inhaled substances varies greatly with the degree of their symptoms. Many patients have a maximal possible response at any given time which cannot be improved by inhaling further bronchodilators although the total inhaled dose required to achieve this maximum varies with the severity of the illness (Gay and Long, 1949; Hume and Gandevia, 1957). The systemic side effects from a given aerosol inhalation may also depend on the clinical state of the patient since they are related to the frequency with which the aerosol has been previously used. Both an increased sensitivity or tachyphylaxis (Robillard *et al.*, 1962) and a decreased response (Paterson *et al.*, 1968) have been described.

The remarkable sensitivity of some patients to bronchodilators was demonstrated by Altounyan (1964) who found that, in a group of his patients with airway obstruction, 90% of the maximum possible response was obtained with an inhaled dose of less than 0·1 mg isoprenaline administered either with a Wright (1958) nebulizer or with a pressurized dispenser. Hume (1969) also stated that 90% of a representative group of asthmatics obtained maximum possible bronchodilation after inhalation of 0·25 mg or less of isoprenaline and that changes in the pulse rate was minimal at this dosage level.

The lack of further benefit obtained by increasing the dose in these circumstances was shown by Cohen and Hale (1965). They found that 0·32 mg isoprenaline was required to produce a significant improvement in their particular group of patients, but that there was no further improvement when the dose was increased from 0·5 mg delivered with a pressurized nebulizer to 5·0 mg given with an intermittent positive pressure breathing apparatus (IPPB). Feinemann and Newell (1963) obtained similar results in patients with chronic bronchitis. They showed that 0·5 mg isoprenaline, delivered by a pressurized nebulizer, was as good as 5 mg delivered by a compressed air apparatus.

While it is clear that excessive dosage is useless and simply increases the risk of untoward side effects, it is not valid to assume that these are best avoided by the use of exceedingly fine sprays since the dose may also be controlled by limiting the duration of the use of the nebulizer or by diluting the solution. Robillard *et al.* (1962) thus found that a Dautrebande (D. 30) spray gave rise to less cardiovascular side effects than a nebulizer producing larger particles and concluded that the D. 30 spray should be used in therapy. The coarser spray delivered about 30–40 times the dose, however, and increased side effects were inevitable. Keighley (1968) compared the response of 12 patients with bronchitis and emphysema to a probable dose of 2·5 mg isoprenaline from a nebulizer producing a majority of particles in the range 1–5 μ diameter with the response to 0·15 mg isoprenaline from a Dautrebande type of generator (mass median diameter probably about 1 μ). The increase in FEV_1 was the same with each type of spray, although there was more tachycardia associated with the nebulizer delivering 2·5 mg isoprenaline. The Dautrebande spray thus produced as much improvement with 0·15 mg isoprenaline as did the coarser spray delivering 2·5 mg. It might be concluded from these results that small particles are more efficient, but Altounyan (1964) had already shown that 0·1 mg of isoprenaline, from a relatively coarse spray, was highly effective in his patients and the experiments of Keighley (1968) may only confirm that excessive dosage is unnecessary and must be avoided. There is no reason at present to assume that this cannot be done by nebulizing more dilute solutions of bronchodilators. The actual number of particles in the cloud is unlikely to be a fundamental factor as far as nebulizer design is concerned since a deficit can be compensated by increasing the number of inhalations. The fact that a few inhalations from a D.30 spray (Dautrebande, 1962) proved to be as effective as 20 or 30 such inhalations may only reflect the extreme sensitivity of a particular group of asthmatic subjects to bronchodilators, and cannot be assumed without further evidence to depend on the number of particles in the cloud.

The site of particle deposition in the lung may be related to the systemic side effects by a further mechanism. Isoprenaline is rapidly detoxicated in sputum (Altounyan, 1964) and also by pharmacological agents in the bronchial wall itself (Patterson *et al.*, 1968). If these mechanisms are only active in certain regions of the airways then access of the drug to the systemic circulation must depend on the deposition pattern of the inhaled particles and hence on their size.

The uniformity of particle size in therapeutic aerosols is probably unimportant. Although the coagulation of particles is more rapid in poly-disperse clouds, this is a minor factor in relation to the concentrations normally employed and there is unlikely to be any benefit in the use of uniform aerosols per se.

The crucial experiment in attempting to determine the effect of particle size must be to examine the results of equal doses of pharmacological compounds deposited in the lung from aerosols containing particles of different sizes. It is important to measure the real dose retained in the body and due allowance must be made for loss of particles in the delivery tubing of the apparatus and for any aerosol exhaled. Simply estimating the loss of fluid from a reservoir may give very misleading results. Although the measurement of the dose of a pharmacological agent deposited in the lung presents severe difficulties the use of radioactive tracers suggested by Patterson *et al.* (1968) should be a valuable technique for this purpose. The pattern of breathing also requires consideration since a deep inhalation results in a further penetration of aerosol into the lung than a shallow inhalation whatever the particle size. This is particularly important in the case of pressurized aerosol dispensers where the whole dose of medicament is released in a few ml of gas (Cohen, 1971).

In comparing the efficiency of different pharmacological compounds it is necessary to establish the minimum dose of each which produces a near maximal bronchodilatation and to assess any side effects at this level of dosage. The agents to be compared must be administered by identical methods. If different techniques are to be used then it may be impossible to distinguish genuine pharmacological effects from those associated with particles of different size.

At present it can only be suggested that bronchodilator aerosols should be fine enough to ensure that little or no particle deposition takes place in the mouth and fauces, and this implies that no particle should be greater than about 10 micron in diameter. Inhalation should be through the mouth rather than via the nose because of the high probability of particle deposition in the latter. Several deep inhalations are more likely to produce an even distribution of particles in the lung than a single breath. The use of intermittent positive pressure breathing apparatus is often used for the administration of aerosols and this is certainly a convenient method of helping patients with airways obstruction to breathe deeply, although there is little evidence that it improves the clinical response.

Humidification of Inhaled Air

The efficient working of the ciliary clearing mechanisms is vital to the integrity of the respiratory tract. The most important factor known to interfere with ciliary action is drying of the mucosa. Inhaled air is normally warmed and humidified in the nose and pharynx so that the lining of the trachea and lower airways is fully moist at all times. This protective mechanism cannot operate if the patient has a tracheotomy, is hyperventilating through the mouth or is breathing very dry anaesthetic gases.

Blanshard (1955) found that the fluid intake of patients had a direct effect on the viscosity of sputum, and experimental dehydration in animals has been shown to interfere with the ciliary clearance mechanism (Bang and Bang, 1961). An adequate fluid intake is thus of the utmost importance in the management of patients with respiratory disease.

Despite such measures, the ciliary and cough mechanism may be overwhelmed by the excessive quantities and sticky nature of sputum in chronic bronchitis and asthma. Sputum retention must be relieved by ensuring that the patient remains as alert as possible and by unremitting help at frequent intervals in assisted coughing. To loosen the sputum, moistening of the inhaled air is also widely used, together with the addition of substances intended to reduce sputum viscosity.

The total amount of water vapour normally added to inhaled air during its passage through the nose, mouth and trachea is of the order of 33 mg per litre, but if the inspired air is completely dry then approximately 44 mg per litre must be added. When the normal air conditioning mechanisms of the upper airways are not functioning then this quantity of water must be artificially added to the inhaled air. For many years the standard technique was to add water vapour to the air by bubbling it through water contained in a Wolf bottle. This method is not very efficient because the passage of dry air through the liquid lowers its temperature and hence the possible moisture content of the air. The only way in which the water content of the air can be further increased using this apparatus is by warming the water reservoir. In this case it is essential to ensure that the reservoir cannot boil dry since this may result in burning of the patient. With this reservation the passage of air through a water bath which is thermostatically controlled is an excellent method of ensuring that the air reaching the patient is both warm and nearly fully saturated with moisture.

Water may also be added in the form of aerosol particles. The old fashioned steam kettle employed this principle and is one example of aerosol therapy which is undoubtedly effective. The response of children with croup may be quite dramatic and the inhalation of warm steam is also comforting in upper respiratory infections in adults, although the addition of substances such as Friar's Balsam or Oil of Eucalyptus has not been shown to add more than a pleasant aroma to the inhalation (Boyd and Sheppard, 1968). There are no data on the sizes of particles in a steam tent and they probably vary with the conditions employed.

The steam tent is cumbersome and it was logical to try spraying the water into the air. Most early methods used unheated aerosols although it is by no means certain that the warm temperature of the older inhalations was an unimportant factor in their effectiveness. It is also difficult to obtain a sufficient quantity of water in such aerosols. Nebulizers can be obtained with a very high water output but this is usually achieved by means of a coarse spray containing very large particles. These large droplets precipitate in the delivery tubing of the apparatus and the patient rarely receives adequate water. The type of nebulizer which delivers a finer spray, such as that described by Wright (1958) has an output of only about 30–40 mgs of water per litre of air. Most of this water will, indeed, be deposited in the patient but it is barely sufficient to supply the basic requirements let alone supply additional moisture. The situation was radically changed by the introduction of ultrasonic nebulizers. These instruments are capable of producing dense clouds of particles containing up to 200 mg per litre. The aerosol is not as fine or as uniform as was originally supposed and the mass median diameter of a representative cloud is about 6 μ (Mercer *et al.*, 1968). Very high concentrations are only available to a patient inhaling directly from the nebulizer and this is clearly impractical for more than a short time. For prolonged use a mist tent is required. The density of the aerosol in such tents is less than that measured at the output of the generator, because of sedimentation of droplets in the delivery tubing or in the tent and because of admixture with dry room air. The total moisture content (droplets and vapour) may be only about 50 to 80 mg of water per litre of air (Doershuk *et al.*, 1968; Wolfsdorf *et al.*, 1969) and the mass median diameter of the particles about 2·8 μ (Wolfsdorf *et al.*, 1969). Since most inhaled particles of this size are deposited in the nose of a sleeping patient the amount reaching the finer airways is likely to be small. Wolfsdorf *et al.* (1969) calculated that only about 200 ml of water was likely to reach the lower respiratory tract of a child in 24 hours of exposure. Whether this is an effective amount in the treatment of such conditions as mucoviscidosis can, of course, be answered only by controlled clinical trials.

An alternative approach to the administration of moisture to the respiratory tract is to saturate the air of the patient's room or ward with various forms of humidifiers. The difficulty of this method again lies in the amount of moisture that the air can hold. A room temperature of about 22°C is normally considered the maximum for comfort but fully saturated air only contains 20 mg of moisture per litre at this temperature. This is only half the amount required to saturate the tidal air at body temperature and the respiratory tract itself must still supply some 20 mg of water per litre of air instead of the normal 33 mg.

Stability of Water Aerosols

There has been, and continues to be, much controversy over the behaviour of water particles in the lung. The tidal air itself is rapidly warmed and humidified in the nose, mouth and pharynx so that it attains body temperature (37°C) before it reaches the bifurcation of the trachea and is nearly fully saturated with moisture at this temperature.

The problem arises as to the stability of water droplets in this inhaled air. This stability is determined by the relationship between the vapour pressure of water at the surface of the droplet and that in the surrounding air. Depending on this ratio water will diffuse towards, or away from, the drop and cause it to change in size. With small droplets the change may take place with great rapidity.

The vapour pressure of water in the lung does not quite correspond to full saturation at the ambient temperature because of the solutes in the fluid lining the alveoli. The alveolar vapour pressure is, in fact, about 46·8 mm Hg while that of pure water at 37°C (body temperature) is about 47·1 mm Hg. The difference appears small but, as will be seen, may be of great importance. The tidal air is warmed and humidified simultaneously in its passage to the alveoli by heat and moisture diffusing from the surface of the mucosa. Since the transfer coefficients of heat and moisture are nearly identical the relative saturation of the air cannot fall appreciably as its temperature rises. However, there is insufficient detailed information at present concerning the pattern of airflow in the upper airway to predict the exact sequence of events, and it is possible that the relative humidity of the tidal air may fall transiently before it reaches equilibrium within the alveoli.

The droplet itself can only acquire heat by conduction from the surrounding air since radiation from the surface of the airway is negligible. However, the vapour pressure of small droplets may be higher than that of the bulk liquid at the same temperature because the curvature of this droplet surface weakens the forces of molecular attraction. The vapour pressure of a 1 μ diameter droplet of pure water and at a temperature of 37°C, for example, is 47·18 mm Hg while that at a plane surface is 47·07 mm Hg. Despite the small size of this difference it produces a characteristic instability in a cloud of particles of mixed sizes. The smaller droplets evaporate and recondense on the larger particles by a process called isothermal distillation. The effect is very sensitive to the size of the particle however, and, at body temperature, the increase in vapour pressure at the surface of a 4 μ diameter droplet is only about 0·03 mm Hg and the theoretical lifetime of such a droplet is very much longer. Solutes in the droplet lower its vapour pressure according to their molecular weight and concentration while contamination of the surface by some chemical substances may also have profound effects.

The behaviour of inhaled water droplets therefore depends upon their size and composition. Droplets of pure water probably evaporate very rapidly indeed. This is likely to be due to the relatively low vapour pressure of the fluid lining the surface of the lung produced by its various solutes or, in the case of droplets of 1 μ in diameter or less, to their surface curvature and its associated effect on vapour pressure. It is often suggested that the rise in temperature of the inhaled air must, in itself, lead to rapid evaporation of the droplets but, as noted, this is not so if the surface of the respiratory tract also adds moisture to the air at the same time, as of course it does. There is great need for direct experimental evidence on this point which is of considerable practical importance, but the technical difficulties are formidable and no work has so far been published. Some indirect information is suggested by Cheyney and Butler (1968) who found that dense aerosols of distilled water caused coughing in both normal subjects and patients with airway obstruction while increased airway resistance was also noted in the latter subjects. It is a matter of common experience that inhaled aerosols of distilled water cause coughing and this is at least some evidence that a fraction of the droplets survive long enough to be deposited in the respiratory tract.

The transfer of moisture from the droplet may be retarded by surface contamination with certain substances. Eisner *et al.* (1960) showed that 0·05–0·2% of a fatty alcohol dispersed in the water could greatly increase the lifetime of a 10 μ diameter droplet in an unsaturated atmosphere, although this method has not received attention in medicine as yet.

Droplets containing dissolved substances absorb or lose water until their vapour pressure is identical with that of the body fluids. For larger particles this will correspond to 0·9 Gm % Saline or 2·5 Gm% propylene glycol, but for droplets as small as 1 micron in diameter a higher concentration would be required. Calculations suggest that the change in size of hypotonic or hypertonic droplets is sufficiently rapid to ensure that they are virtually isotonic before deposition but direct experimental evidence is lacking.

From the practical point of view the difficulties are resolved by using isotonic aerosols whenever it is thought desirable to deposit as much moisture in the respiratory tract as is possible. There is every reason to suppose that such droplets remain unchanged in size and that they are deposited at the appropriate points in the lung according to that size. The exact behaviour of droplets of distilled water or of hypertonic saline and isotonic droplets as small as 1 μ in diameter must remain speculative for the present.

Water droplets evaporate very rapidly when mixed with relatively dry room air as may occur when using a mist tent. This evaporation may be delayed by adding hygroscopic substances to the liquid but it is difficult to see how this can affect the total moisture content (vapour and droplets) of the air in the tent. It may even reduce it because larger particles are more likely to fall out on exposed horizontal surfaces.

Methods of Producing Aerosols

(1) **Air Jet Nebulizers.** The earliest nebulizers were based on the familiar scent spray pattern in which an air jet shatters a continuous liquid supply into separate droplets. The suction effect of the air jet itself maintains the flow of liquid. The cloud has a very wide range of particle sizes and it is usual to place a baffle immediately in front of the jet so that the larger droplets are removed by impaction and drain back into the fluid reservoir. If the baffle is placed very close to the jet then some of the larger drops may be shattered into smaller particles. The air supply may be either a hand bulb, motor pump or gas cylinder. Since the air pressure from a hand bulb is so low the output is correspondingly minute. This is not entirely a disadvantage because at least overdosage is difficult. The liquid lost from the reservoir does not all appear as aerosol particles because some evaporates and saturates the air supply. This may be considerable if the pressure is obtained from a cylinder which contains completely dry gas and the concentration of the remaining substances dissolved in the liquid reservoir of the nebulizer therefore increases with time. The amount of liquid that appears in the aerosol stream depends very much on the design of the baffle system. Nebulizers with a high output achieve this by allowing the larger particles to escape. These larger particles have a strong tendency to deposit in the delivery tubing of the inhalation apparatus and it is problematical as to how much actually reaches the patient. More

efficient baffling produces a fine spray with a correspondingly lower volume content. One of the best patterns is that designed by Wright (1958). The maximum particle diameter in the spray is about 8 μ and the total mass concentration about 30–40 mg of water per litre of air.

A different atomizer was designed by Dautrebande (1962). The larger particles are removed in a series of liquid barriers and the eventual spray is exceedingly fine. The figures for particle size quoted by Dautrebande (1962) refer to the residual crystals after evaporation to dryness of dilute saline aerosols. The size of the original droplets is not stated but they are probably 2 or 3 times larger than the dry crystals. The total number of particles in the cloud is high (up to 20 million per ml) and, although many of the original droplets are between 0·3 to 0·9 μ in diameter (corresponding to sodium chloride crystals 0·1 to 0·34 μ diameter), the mass median diameter (see Chapter 1) may in fact be larger than 1 μ. The total dose delivered by this type of spray is about 20 times less than that of the Wright nebulizer in the same period of use.

(2) **Pressurized Aerosol Dispensers.** Because of their outstanding convenience these dispensers have largely replaced the hand operated nebulizers in recent years. They are small, do not spill and preserve drugs such as isoprenaline indefinitely. The dose is fairly accurately measured.

There are two basic patterns. In one the pharmacological agent is dispersed as a fine dry powder in an inert Freon propellant. When a small volume of the liquid propellant is released it rapidly evaporates to leave the dry particles suspended in air. In the second type of dispenser the agent is dissolved in a solvent such as alcohol and again mixed with propellant. On release both the propellant and alcohol must evaporate before the dry particles are freely suspended in air. The particles in most types are stated by the makers to be less than 5 μ in diameter. However, Patterson *et al.* (1968) found that about 43% of a dose of isoprenaline inhaled from a pressurized dispenser was deposited in the mouth and pharynx. The reputed size of the particles should not result in anything like this deposition in the upper airways. Further evidence that much of the agent in a pressurized aerosol is effectively contained in large particles was found by Kirk (1969) who measured the penetration of the aerosol through a system of glass tubes. The large size of the particles may be because the propellant has insufficient time to evaporate before impaction on the back of the mouth. Another possibility is that several dry particles may be present in a single drop of liquid propellant and that these fail to separate.

Many patients also have difficulty in releasing the dose at the correct time and the particles cannot reach the small airways. More reliable administration by a breath activated release mechanism is described by Cohen (1971). Despite these difficulties there is no doubt that pressurized aerosols have been a tremendous boon to patients and are highly effective in practice.

(3) **Ultrasonic nebulizers.** The outstanding characteristic of these nebulizers is their highly concentrated output of up to 200 mg of water per litre of air which is achieved by means of large numbers of relatively small particles. The size of the particles is not quite so small or as uniform as was originally thought and two reports have shown mass median diameters of about 6 μ with geometric standard deviations of 1·5 to 2·5 (Goddard *et al.*, 1968; Wolfsdorf *et al.*, 1969). The concentration of particles is about 1 or 2 million per cc of air. The ultrasonic energy produced is highly concentrated at the surface of the liquid to be nebulized but there is no evidence that this alters the pharmacological activity of dissolved substances (Goddard *et al.* 1968). Since the size of the particles is related to the frequency of the ultrasonic wave it should be possible to obtain particles of any desired size. This would be of value if it should eventually turn out that the particle size is of real clinical importance. If a patient is inhaling the dense cloud directly from the generator then the solution in the reservoir should be isotonic and should contain 0·9 Gm% NaCl or 2·5% propylene glycol. This will usually prevent coughing but a suitable dilute bronchodilator may also be required for asthmatics. Propylene glycol may be preferred to saline because it is not corrosive to metallic objects and reduces contamination by pseudonomonas organisms (Matthews *et al.*, 1968). For mist tent therapy half strength saline or propylene glycol is probably better because some evaporation takes place in the tent and a weaker solution in the generator makes it likely that the droplets are nearly isotonic when inhaled by the patient.

(4) **Dry particle dispensers.** Some drugs are administered as a dry powder without initial solution in liquids. This is usually because large quantities of a poorly soluble substance are required to achieve a therapeutic effect. Pituitary snuff was once used in this manner.

Disodium Cromoglycate ("Intal") is also prescribed in this way and for the same reasons. The powder contains large particles of an inert compound to improve the running quality of the grains. The active agent in the original powder has 50% by weight in the particle size range of 2–6 μ diameter. However, many of the particles remain aggregated during inhalation and only 1–2 mg out of an original 20 mg are likely to have an aerodynamic size in the range of 2–6 μ. Most of the material is probably deposited at a relatively high level in the respiratory tract (Cox, 1969) but, of course, it cannot be assumed that this is disadvantageous or that better results would be obtained by using smaller airborne particles.

(5) **Uniform aerosol generators.** A method of producing aerosols in which the particles are all the same size was described by Walton and Prewett (1949). The liquid to be nebulized is fed on to the centre of a spinning disc at a rate of about 1 ml per minute. The disc has a diameter of about 2·5 cm and is driven by compressed air or by an electric motor at speeds of the order of 100,000 rpm. Particles of more than one size are produced but they can be separated into uniform clouds. Low concentrations of particles of much more uniform size may be obtained by means of liquids fed through capillaries vibrated at high frequencies.

These generators are not used for clinical purposes but have considerable value as research instruments because the particle size can be controlled between narrow limits. The behaviour of particles of a single size can thus be studied.

Conclusions

The clinical use of aerosols has developed in a random fashion. Potent agents are administered with very little knowledge as to the performance of the delivery apparatus, or even of its desired performance. The complexity of the various factors which must be considered suggests that theoretical calculations should be viewed with considerable caution and that only controlled assessment of the therapeutic response can be accepted as a genuine measure of their true value.

References

Altounyan, R. E. C. (1964), "Variation of Drug Action on Airway Obstruction in Man." *Thorax*, **19**, 406.

Bang, B. G. and Bang, F. B. (1961), "Effect of Water Deprivation on Mucous Flow." *Proc. Soc. Exptl. Biol. Med.*, **106**, 46.

Blanshard, G. (1955), "The Viscosity of Sputum." *Arch. Middx. Hosp.*, **5**, 222.

Boyd, E. M. and Sheppard, E. P. (1968), "The Effect of Steam Inhalation of Volatile Oils on the Output and Composition of Respiratory Tract Fluid." *J. Pharmacol. Exp. Ther.*, **163**, 250.

Cheney, F. W. and Butler, J. "The Effects of Ultrasonically-produced Aerosols on Airway Resistance in Man." *Anesthesiology*, **29**, 1099.

Cohen, A. A. and Hale, F. C. (1965), "Comparative Effects of Isoproterenol Aerosols on Airway Resistance in Obstructive Pulmonary Diseases." *Amer. J. Med. Sc.*, **249**, 309.

Cohen, B. M. (1971), "Metered Aerosols of Bronchodilator Drugs in Clinical Trials." *Thorax*, **26**, 316.

Cox, J. S. G. (1969), "Correspondence." *Brit. Med. J.*, **3**, 177.

Dautrebande, L. (Publ. 1962), *Microaerosols*. New York: Academic Press.

Doershuk, C. F., Matthews, L. W., Gillespie, C. T., Lough, M. D. and Spector, S. (1968), "Evaluation of Jet Type and Ultrasonic Nebulisers in Mist Tent Therapy for Cystic Fibrosis." *Pediatrics*, **41**, 723.

Eisner, H. S., Quince, B. W. and Slack, C. (1960), "The Stabilization of Water Mists by Insoluble Monolayers." *Disc. Faraday Soc.*, **80**, 86.

Ephraim, A. (1930), "Uber die Bedeutung der Bronchoskopie für die innere medizin." *Berl. Klin. Schnschr.*, **109**, 44.

Fenmann, L. and Newell, D. J. (1963), "Isoprenaline in the Treatment of Chronic Bronchitis." *Brit. J. Dis. Chest.*, **57**, 140.

Gay, L. N. and Long, J. W. (1949), "Clinical Evaluation of Isopropyl-epinephrine in Management of Bronchial Asthma." *J. Amer. Med. Ass.*, **139**, 452.

Goddard, R. F., Mercer, T. T., O'Neill, P. X. F., Flores, R. L. and Sanchez, R. (1968), "Output Characteristics and Clinical Efficacy of Ultrasonic Nebulizers." *J. Asthma. Res.*, **5**, 355.

Graeser, J. B. and Rowe, A. H. (1935), "Inhalation of Epinephrine for the Relief of Asthmatic Symptoms." *J. Allergy*, **6**, 415.

Hume, K. M. and Gandevia, B. (1957), "Forced Expiratory Volumes Before and After Isoprenaline." *Thorax*, **12**, 276.

Hume, K. M. H. (1969), "Treating Asthma." *Brit. Med. J.*, **1**, 515.

Keighley, J. F. (1968), "Response to Sympathomimatic Aerosols of Differing Particle Size in Subjects with Chronic Bronchitis." *Amer. Rev. Resp. Dis.*, **98**, 879.

Kirk, W. F. (1969), "An in vitro Method for Comparison of the Efficiency o Aerosols from Various Pressurized Inhalers in the Penetration of Airways." *Ceskoslov. Farm.*, **18**, 142.

Matthews, L. W., Doershuk, C. F., Miller, S. T., Pittman, S. and Lough, M. (1968), "Mist Tent Therapy of Cystic Fibrosis." *J. Asthma Res.*, **5**, 267.

Mercer, T. T., Goddard, R. F. and Flores, R. L. (1968), "Output Characteristics of Three Ultrasonic Nebulisers." *Ann. Allergy*, **24**, 18.

Nadel, J. A., Corn, M., Swl, S., Flesch, J. and Graf, P. (1967), "Location and Mechanism of Airway Constriction after Inhalation of Histamine Aerosol and Inorganic Sulfate Aerosol." In *Inhaled Particles and Vapours* II. Ed. C. N. Davies. London: Pergamon Press.

Patterson, J. W., Conolly, M. E., Davies, D. S. and Dollery, C. T. (1968), "Isoprenaline Resistance and the Use of Pressurized Aerosols in Asthma." *Lancet*, **12**, 426.

Robillard, E., Pine, Ch. le and Dautrebande, L. (1962), "Influence of Particle Size on Systemic Effects After Breathing Potent Medicated Aerosols." *Can. Med. Ass. J.*, **86**, 362.

Segal, M. S. (1962), "Inhalation Therapy for Chronic Lung Disease." *Anesthesiology*, **23**, 513.

Walton, W. H. and Prewett, W. C. (1949), "The Production of Sprays and Mists of Uniform Drop Size by Means of Spinning Disc Type Sprayers." *Proc. Physical Soc. B.*, **62**, 341.

Wolfsdorf, J., Swift, D. L. and Avery, M. W. (1969), "Mist Therapy Reconsidered, an Evaluation of the Respiratory Deposition of Labelled Water Aerosols Produced by Jet and Ultrasonic Nebulizers." *Pediatrics*, **43**, 799.

Wright, B. M. (1958), "A New Nebulizer." *Lancet*, **2**, 24.

INDEX